Who Gets to
Choose
?

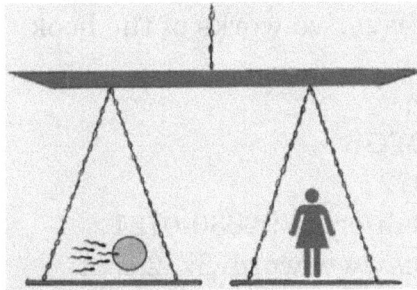

The Moral, Legal and, yes,
Religious case for
Reproductive Choice

T. F. Barans

Word Wizards, Escondido, California

Published by:
Word Wizards®
P.O. Box 300721
Escondido, California 92030-0721
website: http://www.wordwiz72.com

ISBN Number (print edition): 978-0-944363-20-1
ISBN Number (e-book edition): 978-0-944363-21.8

CONTENTS

★

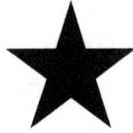

INTRODUCTION

W ho gets to choose?

Who owns a woman's body?

Who should get to make decisions over the most private aspects of a woman's body?

For millennia of human history, men dominated all aspects of the economic, political and personal lives of women. They created social and moral traditions that they insisted were decreed by God himself. And their god was definitely a *"him*self" — a very angry and misogynistic "himself." They enforced total control over women.

In the nineteenth century, women began to exert pressure for political equality and demanded the right to vote. In the twentieth century, women expanded their political influence to include the right to hold public office. They pushed for true economic equality, demanding more equal opportunities in the workplace and more equal access to all aspects of employment opportunity and advancement.

With the advent of contraception, women beat back resistance from religious conservatives to popularize new resources for true reproductive independence and freedom on a scale previously enjoyed only by men, who could engage in sexual intimacy without concern of unwanted or unplanned pregnancies.

With the taste of sexual freedom afforded by the "pill," women began to push the boundaries even further. In instances where new resources failed to prevent unwanted pregnancy, whether by product defect or user error, women decided they no longer wished to revert to the days when their lifestyle choices could be threatened by a pregnancy they did not want.

Women decided that the option to *prevent* unwanted pregnancy, as empowering as that was, was not enough. They also wanted to be able to reverse unwanted outcomes after the fact. They wanted to be able to undo any unwanted pregnancy.

They wanted the right to legal abortion.

They wanted the right to **CHOOSE**.

Who gets to choose?

Women decided they wanted it to be themselves, and not someone else. Their bodies; their choices.

But there would be a backlash. Men had held all the power for thousands of years. And some men, often joined by women who had acquiesced to their domination, felt threatened by a loss of that power. And in the name of "tradition" and "that's the way it's always been" and "God said so," they intended to stand their controlling ground.

Somehow, these traditionalist men, backed up by acquiescent women, felt they had the right to make decisions about the most private parts of women's bodies during the brief period of months that such bodies are occupied by pre-sentient embryonic and fetal life.

Ironically, these same men who claim to stand up for the "rights" of embryonic and fetal cell tissue while inside women's bodies can callously invade other nations and shoot or bomb children and pregnant women and think nothing of the embryonic and fetal lives they destroy.

And somehow the defense of embryonic or fetal cell tissue that was so important when it was insentient and pre-conscious while inside a woman's body, becomes less deserving of protection once it is no longer inside that female body that needs to be controlled.

Many of the same men who demand that women carry pregnancies to childbirth demonstrate utter disregard for the lives of those children after they have been born, while they are too young and small and helpless to be of productive use for generating the monetary profits they covet above all else. Such men are eager to eliminate funding and resources for education and support services for actual children who have been born, yet express a profound interest in controlling women's private lives right up until the point of such births.

Such hypocritical double standards clearly demonstrate the reality that their only true motive in trying to micromanage the most private aspects of women's lives is solely domination and control. They seek to enforce subservience over a population that they feel they are entitled to control.

To a great extent, this reflects long histories of patriarchal, male-dominated religious traditions dictating that men should be masters over women, and control all aspects of their lives, from the financial to the sexual to the very control over their reproductive freedoms and the most private parts of their bodies.

Over the millennia, this domination — rooted in its religious origins — has been expressed in many forms.

Nathaniel Hawthorne's classic, *The Scarlet Letter,* introduces us to Hester Prynne, a young wife who becomes pregnant while her husband is away in Europe and who could not possibly have fathered her pregnancy.

Because the pregnancy so obviously is not the result of marital relations as required by their strict legalistic erotophobic tradition of moralistic Massachusetts of the 17th Century Puritans, Hester is found guilty of not only a mortal sin, but also a violation of criminal law.

Her punishment, according to their Bible-based law, should be death, despite her stubborn (or stoic) refusal to identify her child's father. But a compassionate pastor argues for mercy and, instead, the punishment is reduced to being publicly shamed and humiliated by being forced to wear a prominent scarlet letter "**A**" for adultery on her chest and to be shunned, living on the outskirts of town with her baby. Not surprisingly, it turns out that the pastor ends up being revealed as the child's father. He is racked by guilt and torment over his transgression, but he otherwise escapes formal punishment.

Oh well, boys will be boys.

While adultery is still looked down upon today, in our times no one would consider it to be a criminal violation, but rather a personal matter to be addressed privately. Today we would find the idea of public shaming or public punishment for a private moral offense to be primitive and barbaric. Even allowing for increasing acceptance of open adultery as highlighted by the *Ashley Madison* phenomenon, the vast majority who still disapprove of such infidelity and betrayal would consider it a private matter, not a matter of public interference.

Yet there remain some among us, the latter-day Puritans, who do still seek to use the full force of criminal law to impose their moral choices on women, and women who resist find themselves subject to efforts at public shaming.

A woman who gets pregnant but decides she does not wish to have her body occupied against her will for the next nine months, and who chooses a legal, safe, medically-supervised abortion to terminate that unwanted pregnancy, finds herself subjected to public shaming, "sidewalk counseling," being yelled at in public places, possibly the object of online persecution and having private personal information made public and otherwise publicly humiliated, harassed and intimidated.

Even public figures who openly advocate the right of women to control their own bodies are often intimidated. In the media and entertainment industries, for example, there are many who speak out in support of women's reproductive rights. Yet in the many movies, television programs and other media presentations they offer, they will eagerly glorify pregnancy or wrestling with the choice of whether or not to keep an unintended pregnancy if the woman decides to carry the pregnancy to term, but they almost never show, and certainly not in any positive light, someone actually going through the difficult choice to end an unwanted pregnancy even though going through with that decision is a very real part of the very real lives of tens of thousands of women every year and often represents difficult and morally-courageous decisions of conscience.

Women who boldly and openly make a choice not to complete pregnancies they do not want are looked down upon and shunned, to the point where even those in the media are intimidated from backing up their stated pro-choice views with more tangible expressions through their art.

The Scarlet Letter is still alive and well.

Today that large, red "A" stands for **ABORTION**.

Being *pro choice* means supporting a woman's right to make medical and personal decisions about the most private parts of her own body regarding sexuality and reproduction.

In the case of pregnancy, it means the right of a woman to be able to choose whether or not to use contraception (and what kind) and, when a pregnancy occurs, to decide if she wishes to continue the pregnancy or not and, if so, on what terms.

Empowering Women — Positive Objectives

This book does recognize the need for resistance against those who would hold women back or return to dark days of past centuries when men dominated women, but it is not ultimately a book that dwells on the negative.

This book is fundamentally **positive** and **optimistic** in its outlook. This book is about **empowerment**, **advancement** and **opportunity**.

Women have made tremendous gains in the past 150 years, but there remains much more to achieve in order to attain real, true equality and personal freedom. *This book encourages and looks ahead towards those continued gains.*

And sometimes that means standing up against those who not only object to such further advancement, but also seek to roll it back to the moral dark ages of the past.

Pro Life or Pro Choice or Pro Abortion

One point that requires clarification in advance is the use of terminology. We hear terms such as "pro-life" or "pro-choice" employed by each side in the struggle for true personal equality.

Those who oppose women's further advancement and seek to move backward rather than forward like to call themselves "pro life," because they support forcibly keeping embryos and fetuses alive. Yet many of the same proponents of forced pregnancy also support the death penalty, aggressive military action including wars and even forced pregnancy in cases where it could threaten the life of a pregnant woman. And, as already noted, they do not support interventions to save the quality of life of an embryo or fetus once it is actually born and no longer inside a woman's body. As a result, their use of the term "pro life" seems to be a clear case of false advertising. This book will not accommodate such inaccurate and misleading terminology and will refer to those who oppose a woman's right to make personal choices about her own body in more accurate terms. This book will refer to them as "anti-choice."

To be "pro-**choice**" means that, if a pregnancy occurs that is unwanted, the woman — in consultation with whatever medical, family, counseling or other advisors *she **alone** chooses* — decides whether to continue the pregnancy to term and keep the resulting child, continue the pregnancy to term and adopt the child out, or not to continue the pregnancy (i.e., whether or not to have an abortion).

Those who favor the right of women to make their own choices about their own bodies have a much stronger case in calling themselves "pro choice." They support choice. Period. Whatever the choice —

whether to carry a pregnancy to term and keep the resulting baby, or carry to term and adopt out, or to not complete the unwanted pregnancy — those of us who are pro-choice believe it is the woman, and only the woman, who should be empowered to make such choices.

Some of those who oppose empowering women with the right to make their own choices about their bodies ignore the full range of possible choices we believe should be available to women and, insist that anyone who supports the right of a woman to choose to abort an unwanted pregnancy must really be "pro abortion," not "pro choice."

But since the right to choose includes the full array of choices, and not just abortion, that is an inaccurate description that reflects either a lack of understanding or an intentional misrepresentation of others' views.

Now, I don't doubt that there are some who promote abortion, such as the anti-choice forced abortions of China and its "one child" policy that curtails women's right to choose to carry more than one pregnancy to term and mandates required forced abortion of any pregnancy that violates that very restrictive limitation. Those who support policies requiring mandatory abortion could accurately be said to be *pro abortion,* but that does not apply to those who support true reproductive choice and who find such policies invasive, abhorrent and a brutal act of oppression that tramples women's reproductive rights.

To those of us who are truly pro-*choice,* those who support mandatory forced abortion are as reprehensible as those who support mandatory forced pregnancies, enforced by Big Intrusive Government micromanaging the private medical choices that religious tyrants wish to mandate. Those who support government-mandated forced abortion (such as in Communist China) and those who support government-enforced (such as religious conservatives) represent the same mentality of supporting big government intrusion in dictating their choices over women's bodies. The only difference is that they want their big intrusive government to enforce different choices.

In contrast, it is my experience that when people are referred to as being "pro-abortion," more commonly it is a reference to supporting the *right* to choose an abortion, or any other choice, such as to choose to adopt out or to choose to carry and keep — whatever *choice* the *woman* wants. The support the woman's right to make whichever choice among all options she wants, and they do not promote, encourage or otherwise push any specific option, including abortion. Therefore, they are no more correctly labeled "pro-abortion" than they are "pro-adoption" or "pro-parenting" since they support all of these options equally, depending on what each woman decides is right for herself.

For example, some have called me "pro abortion" which is not true. I promote the *right* to make that *or any other choice,* whether that be to carry a pregnancy to term and keep the child that is born, carry a pregnancy to term and let other parents adopt it, or *not* to carry the pregnancy to term.

My own personal *opinion* is that abortion is a remedial response to an unfortunate and unwanted situation, and is better prevented but, if needed, remedial treatment to correct the unwanted condition should be available.

Similarly, I believe that a root canal is a remedial response to an unfortunate condition of oral disease, but that even if the person has poor eating and hygiene habits or preventive care fails, patients should have the right to choose that treatment option rather than, say, full removal of the diseased tooth.

I would not call myself "pro-*root canal*," but I do support the right to that treatment option, even though it kills millions of biologically autonomous living creatures (bacteria) occupying and infecting the neural canals of diseased dental tissue, because I happen to believe that a single sentient human **person**, who happens to be the owner of that particular mouth, is the only one who has the right to make that decision.

Legality and Morality Differentiated

In discussing the issue of abortion, there are two distinct aspects to consider: the **moral** issue and the **legal** issue. It is possible to hold the view that abortion is not *moral,* yet not subscribe to the view that it should be subject to regulation as a matter of law. For example, many believe it to be a moral transgression — a sin — for two unmarried consenting adults to engage in sexual intimacy, but almost

15

no one would think it should be criminalized as a matter of law (we've come a long way from the days of Hester Prynne and the Puritans).

In the chapters that follow, we will examine the *moral* issues and the *legal* issues as the separate dimensions that they are.

We will then also discuss, as a subset to the moral issue for those who are religious believers, the misguided origins of religious prohibitions against abortion based on misinterpretations of religious texts by those who, perhaps in their moralistic Puritanical zeal, may even distort those religious texts intentionally.

Following the presentations of core **moral**, **legal** and **religious** issues in reproductive choice, we will then examine some additional issues in reproductive choice that are often raised, such as late term abortion, parental consent, abortion resulting from rape or incest, the role Planned Parenthood is perceived to play in the subject of abortion, and other issues. We will consider some of the arguments made by those who oppose empowering women to control their own bodies and how, when we go deeper than just the surface, superficial slogans, the arguments offered actually work against those who raise them.

Additionally, we will consider how some of the issues and factors often perceived as being specific to the subject of abortion also influence other contemporary moral and social issues of broader public policy, such as thoughts about human cloning (either for reproduction or, more commonly, as a source of embryonic stem cells for autologous organ regeneration), other embryonic stem cell research and therapies, in-vitro fertilization (very controversial and opposed by religious conservatives when first introduced) and embryonic screening to avoid genetic disorders.

While many see the issue of a woman's right to control her own body as a single specific issue, in reality the issue of a woman's right to choose abortion arises out of other issues of control and domination and leads to how we address other public policy, social and moral issues.

The question begins and ends with control of women's bodies and women's own rights of autonomous bodily sovereignty and self-determination.

Ultimately the question is not only whose body it is but: **Whose Gets to Choose**?

T. F. Barans
San Diego, California

1

Moral Issues:
Life vs. Personhood

The first and most basic question in the issue of reproductive rights is the moral question. Apart from any question of whether abortion should be legal or illegal, the first issue is whether or not it is a violation of ethical or moral standards.

It is extremely possible, and often the case, that something can be judged to be unethical or immoral but does not rise to the level of requiring public policy intervention.

At one time, governments decided that adultery — the violation of marital vows — was not only immoral, but should be prohibited as a matter of law. Violators were punished, often put to death. The

American writer Nathaniel Hawthorne wrote a scathing critique of such policies in his classic masterpiece, *The Scarlet Letter*. And in his famous classic, the "guilty" heroine Hester Prynne was granted mercy, and received an unusual public shaming — the wearing of a scarlet letter "**A**" sewn to her front of her blouse — in lieu of being put to death.

Yet today, we can look at adultery, which many would still consider a violation of ethical or moral values, to be a private matter of personal relationships, not something that should be enforced as a legislated mandate enforced by criminal penalties. Few in our time would consider it appropriate to be enforced as a matter of criminal law.

In the same way, we can look at the matter of abortion and say that, even if some may consider it to be morally wrong, it could be a private matter of personal belief and opinion, and not a matter to be governed as a matter of criminal law.

But the question of whether or not abortion is ethical or moral is really the first issue that must be addressed. *If the choice to abort an unwanted pregnancy **is not even a moral offense in the first place**,* then even the stated basis for dealing with it as a legal issue — a matter of public policy — becomes moot.

That which some consider morally wrong — what some might call a "sin" — may or may not rise to the level of being legislatively mandated. But *if something is **not even wrong to begin with**,* then any talk of outlawing it becomes irrelevant.

We will deal with the legal issues in the next chapter, and the religious issue in the chapter after that, but if we can resolve the issue at the level of the moral question — if there is nothing wrong with abortion in the first place — then that should be enough to settle the matter out of hand.

In discussing the moral aspects of the issue, we will defer the religious question for now. For those who have strong religious views, their moral views are largely rooted in those religious beliefs, often with complex moral questions being reduced to "because God says so." But because any adequate examination the religious aspect is so extensive, and is not relevant to non-believers or others who want to see moral questions addressed based on inherent issues of right and wrong, we have reserved that for a later chapter all its own.

In that later chapter, we will demonstrate that careful, objective, context-based examination of even the religious issue takes that away from the religious conservatives.

So, is there even anything morally or ethically wrong with allowing a woman to have reproductive control over her own body?

Human Life vs. Being a Human Person

For many who oppose abortion on moral grounds, the issue seems obvious. Life begins at "conception" (the fertilization of egg by sperm) and taking an "innocent" human life is "murder."

Their view: Human life begins at fertilization. The newly-created embryo is a human being. A person.

21

To kill it is the moral equivalent of murder. Seems simple. Straightforward. Obvious. In the words of Dr. Raymond Dennehy, referring to the prenatal uterine content, that "This creature is produced by a human father and a human mother. If it's not a human being, what is it?" (Los Angeles Times, 2-23-2010)

But there is far more to the issue of when a human person begins to exist. The issue consists of much more than simplistically reducing it to the equation: HUMAN LIFE = HUMAN PERSON

The problem for those who equate *human life* with being a *human person* is that those who make this assertion do not apply it consistently to all *human life*. Exactly the same could be said of a human egg or a human sperm *before* fertilization.

Sperms and eggs are produced by human parents.
Sperms and eggs are alive.
Sperms and eggs are human life.

Yeah, yeah, I know — they have not fully achieved the combined genetic status.

But sperms and eggs are **alive**.
Sperms and eggs are of the **human** species.
Sperms and eggs are **human life**.

To say that being a human person depends on whether they have 23 or 46 chromosomes concedes the issue of "human life" and imposes a qualification on when LIFE becomes a PERSON.

To say that it is the number of chromosomes that determines personhood is to acknowledge the recognition that **human life is *not the issue*** — that something more than being *alive* and of the *human species* is necessary for human *life* to become a human *person*.

In any case, basing *personhood* on the number of chromosomes instead of being *alive* gets a bit dicey. If 46 chromosomes is what makes you a person, is it okay to abort a fetus with Turner's syndrome (45 chromosomes) or Down's syndrome (47 chromosomes)? At what number do you draw the line? And why is *this* purely arbitrary standard (a number of chromosomes) a valid basis for saying that some human *life* is a person and other human life is not?

In any case, to say that being a human person requires the human sperm (alive) and the human egg (alive) to combine in order to be a person is to say that human *life* is not the issue at all. It is the combination. Or the chromosomes. Or something, but not life itself.

They can't have it both ways. They can't say it is about "human life" and then make it about combinations of human lives (that were already alive before they combined) or numbers of chromosomes or heartbeats or whatever.

The old cliché that "human life begins at conception" is patently false. No one seriously believes that a human sperm or human egg capable of becoming a future person is either not alive or that it is not of the human species.

The real issue is not human *life* but when that life becomes a *person,* or else you must include sperms and eggs.

As to when human *life* becomes a human *person,* there are many opinions on when this occurs:

When the egg is created or when the sperm is created (when *life* begins).

When the egg and sperm join.

When cell differentiation begins.

When the blastocyst becomes implanted in the uterus to begin the pregnancy.[*]

When a fetal heartbeat commences.

When there is the onset of measurable EEG brain waves (which occurs at about 24-25 weeks; middle of 2nd trimester, as differentiated from routine electrical cell activity in all cells, including sperms and eggs).[†]

When there is actual sentient human consciousness.

---

[*] For anyone who questions that, apart from the question of either life or personhood, that uterine implantation is the point at which the *pregnancy* beings, I would suggest they look at a woman holding a Petri dish with newly fertilized zygotes prior to implantation for in-vitro fertilization. Prior to that zygote being inserted, no one would say that the woman is pregnant. But afterward, everyone would agree that she is pregnant.

[†] Sources from peer-reviewed science on onset of EEG brain waves at 24-25 weeks of pregnancy:

According to Bergstrom, R.M. 1986, Development of EEG and Unit Electrical Activity of the Brain during Ontogeny, In L.J. Jilek and T. Stanislaw (Eds.), "Ontogenesis of the Brain," Prague: University of Karlova Press

Morowitz, Harold J. and Trefil, James S. 1994, "The Facts of Life," Oxford University Press, a study of brainwaves in fetuses younger than 25 weeks, which included fetuses from 59 days old (8.5 weeks) to 158 days old (22.5 weeks), there were no brain waves seen before 25 weeks, although electrical (neural) activity was present (electrical activity is present in ALL cells, including sperms/eggs).

When the fetus emerges from inside the most private part of a woman's body to begin its separate, autonomous experience with the surrounding environment.

At which of these milestones does human *life* become a human *person?*

The answer is a matter of opinion and values.

Some take the Biblical standard: when the new life is BORN and takes its first breath (Gen 2:7).

So many *opinions?* Whose *opinion* counts?

As long as it is inside the most private part of a woman's body, only that woman has the right to make that decision in each situation.

It is *her opinion* and *her opinion only* that matters.

Beginnings and ends. There should be some reasonable inverse correlation between the definition of the end of life and the definition of the beginning of life. The definition of the end of life is the cessation of measurable EEG brain waves, at which point organs can be removed for donation.

Thus, my own preference is to apply the exact inverse of the end of life to the beginning of life: since the cessation of measurable EEG brain waves confirms the fact of death at the end of life, we cannot say there is a human person before the onset of measurable EEG brain waves. There may be human life, but it cannot be considered a human *person*. The same standard for the *end* of life can be reciprocated to delineate the minimum standard for what can be considered the *beginning* of life.

But that is *my opinion* for myself. I do not impose it on anyone else.

Again, to say that anything other than the fact of being alive and of the human species, whether it be the number of chromosomes, a beating heart, the onset of measurable EEG brain waves, the onset of full conscious sentience or biological autonomy at the time of birth, is to acknowledge the recognition that something more than being alive and of the human species is necessary for human *life* to become a human *person*.

In any case, if one believes that **human life** is the standard, then it becomes incumbent on them to offer their specific proposals for ensuring that every **human sperm cell** and every **human ovum** — each a unique and individual **human life** — never be allowed to die unfertilized because, according the standard of being purely **pro-life:**

Menstruation is murder.
Ejaculation is genocide.

Menstruation washes away a formerly living ovum cell that was allowed to wantonly die unfertilized.

Masturbation washes away hundreds of thousands of formerly living sperm cells that were allowed to wantonly die unfertilized.

Each human egg or sperm was alive, or it would not be capable of being fertilized.

Each human egg or sperm was, by definition, of the human species.

Each was a HUMAN LIFE.

Any person who claims that all "life" is inherently sacred and must be protected by force of statutory legal mandate, must be prepared to offer their suggestions for what policies they propose to ensure that no human egg or sperm ever be allowed to die unfertilized.

Any person who does not consider each egg and sperm, before fertilization, a human person must admit that the standard for defining a human *person* is *not mere life,* but requires something else.

Since I do not know of anyone who supports the standard of taking action to ensure that no human egg or human sperm — each a unique human *life* — ever be allowed to die unfertilized, it is safe to say that no one, regardless of what labels they adopt, is truly "pro-life" when it comes to protecting the life of the pre-born.

And it should be pointed out that, while the cessation of measurable EEG brain waves is the standard for determining the end of life, EEG brain waves are not the same as full sentience or consciousness. EEG brain waves are the minimal standard for mental activity. A person can be asleep or unconscious or even in a vegetative state and still have quite active EEG brain wave activity.

On the end of life, the cessation of EEG brain waves is the ultimate standard. Once the minimum threshold for mental activity has ended, there is no more meaningful life, even if other cell activity has not all shut down completely yet.

At the opposite extreme, the onset of EEG brain waves is the barest *minimum* standard for determining the onset of human personhood. At the first moment that EEG brain waves flicker to life, there is far less actual sentience or consciousness than in a fish or a lizard or a mouse.

Sure, if we want to play it utterly safe, just as we do at the end of life, that is absolutely a very safe standard. But even at this point there is nothing remotely resembling real thought, real consciousness, real feeling, real experience, or anything close to that. In contrast, by the time an actual baby has been born, it does have all of those capabilities. It has real thoughts, real consciousness, real feelings and the beginning of real experiences. They may be at a very early beginning stage of development, but they are all there.

The book *Extro•Dynamics,* by Douglas Dunn, is an excellent resource that discusses at length the nature of human sentience and consciousness as the basis for human personhood and the foundation from which our moral and ethical standards are derived and the starting point from which social dynamics and human interactions occur.

Value derives from the process of sentient interaction of consciousness with the surrounding environment as it e**VALU**ates that which it encounters and experiences. And the ultimate in value is the encounter and experience of one sentient consciousness with other sentient consciousnesses, as the inherent process of value that originates in each interacts with and builds upon the inherent value of all the other sentient consciousnesses, in a process in which the sum is greater than the parts.

The concept of *Extro•Dynamics* ultimately leads to a beautiful protocol of human interactions based on empathy and compassion that could not exist in the absence of these human qualities — these very human qualities that exist in babies, toddlers, children, teenagers, adults and seniors but which do not exist in sperm cells, egg cells, embryos or first trimester fetuses.

This is not to say that sperm cells, egg cells, embryos or first trimester fetuses are not capable of having value. Lacking sentience or consciousness of their own, they do not have inherent, intrinsic value. But if the woman whose body they occupy wants them, they may have great value. But it is not their own inherent value; it is value derived via the consciousness of the sentient being that cherishes them. And on the contrary, if the pregnancy is unwanted, there is no inherent value, only pain that only the woman can choose to remediate.

Embryo / Fetus vs. Human Person

Some comparisons of similarities and differences in organisms of HUMAN LIFE:

Is a one-celled human life form?
Ovum: YES.
Sperm: YES.
Newly-fertilized embryo: YES.
Newborn baby: NO

Has measurable EEG brain waves?
Ovum: NO.

Sperm: NO.
Newly-fertilized embryo NO.
Newborn baby: YES

Has actual feelings and sentience?
Ovum: NO.
Sperm: NO.
Newly-fertilized embryo: NO.
Newborn baby: YES

Can be frozen, stored for years, and revived?
Ovum: YES.
Sperm: YES.
Newly-fertilized embryo: YES.
Newborn baby: NO

Is biologically autonomous (not dependent 24/7 on a SPECIFIC non-transferable caregiver)?
Ovum: NO.
Sperm: NO.
Newly-fertilized embryo: NO.
Newborn baby: YES

Sperm / Egg   Embryo / Fetus   Newborn Baby

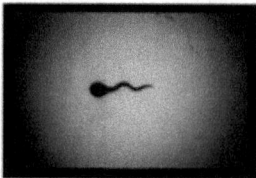

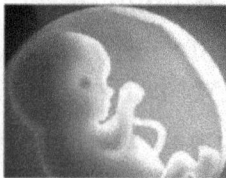

Species: Human
Status: Alive
No Sentience
Not biologically autonomous
No EEG brain waves
Human Life

Species: Human
Status: Alive
No Sentience
Not biologically autonomous
No EEG brain waves
Human Life

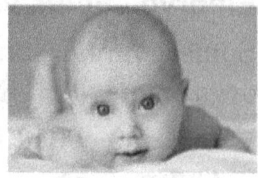

Species: Human
Status: Alive
Fully Sentient & conscious
Biologically autonomous
Measurable EEG brain waves
Human PERSON

If "abortion is murder" ("killing" one pre-sentient, pre-conscious "life"), then menstruation — allowing an pre-fertilized human life to die — is also murder, and ejaculation — allowing hundreds of thousands of human lives to die — is genocide.

The egg and sperm are *human life* before fertilization. A child that has actually been born is a *human person* after birth.

Conservatives show no interest in protecting the *human life* of eggs and sperms before they are in the woman's womb, nor are they willing to provide food or housing to children who have actually been born, but are living in poverty through no fault of their own. The *only* time conservatives show any interest in human life of anyone other than themselves is while it is occupying the most private part of a woman's body. Thus, the only viable conclusion is that it is about controlling women, and has nothing to do with the "sanctity of life."

An *embryo* is no more equal to a *baby* than an *acorn* is to an *oak*. Each has the *potential* to become the actuality of the other. It is no more equal to an ensouled human *person* than a house being built is equal to a completed home with people living in it.

If you mix a batch of blue paint and a batch of yellow paint, you get a new batch of paint: green. But the paint existed before it became green; it was just changed or adapted into a new phase. But before that joining they were all paint. The origin of that batch of green paint began in the batches of yellow and blue paint that formed it. If there were

31

some kind of hazardous chemical wrongly found in the green paint, you can bet that it would be traced back to either the yellow or the blue paint and clearly it would have to be said that the green paint is a continuation of the blue and yellow that came together to form it, though we would all agree that a substantive and important change has occurred. However, in all cases, the blue paint or the yellow paint or the green paint, would still be paint. Not a painting or work of art, but just paint. All of them would have the *potential* to become a painting (or perhaps just be used to paint a fence).

This is not to say that a fertilized egg is not a genetically-uniquely piece of human tissue. A human being is much more than the mere existence of **life**. Insects and bacteria have *life* and uniquely individual DNA. Each is an autonomous, living individual. Is it a sin to get immunizations that kill *millions* of individual lives? Or to use insecticides, or to unnecessarily kill and eat sentient, biologically autonomous birds and mammals non-vegetarians butcher to satisfy their lust for more fat in their arteries?

To be a human *person* is more than merely being *alive*. It is more than merely having human chromosomes and human DNA. It is a combination of life, human genetics, consciousness and sufficient autonomy that it can live apart from its biological mother, even if it still requires someone to be a caregiver, as long as the person is capable of doing so *willingly,* by *choice.*

Trying to equate a *born human person* to a one-celled organism is *dehumanizing* and is just one more example of how religious conservatives seek to minimize the equality, dignity and value of women.

What if your Mother had aborted?

A typical question often thrown out by anti-choice extremists is, "What if your mother had chosen to abort? You wouldn't be here."

While that is undoubtedly true, it does nothing to differentiate the value of a human fetus from that of a human sperm cell or a human egg cell.

How far back do you go?

I can always turn the question back to them and ask, "What if your mother hadn't been 'in the mood' the night you were just a gleam in your father's eye?" Once again, the "logic" of the conservatives' silly question can apply every bit as much to human egg cells or sperm cells before fertilization as to their status afterward. If taken seriously, it leads yet again to the conclusions that, by their standard, every time a woman produces an egg cell or a man produces a sperm cell, if that sperm or egg cell — each a unique human life — is allowed to die unfertilized, it is the moral equivalent of murder.

The absurdity immediately becomes obvious.

But beyond that, the extremists' choices of examples of who might not be here if their mothers had chosen to abort is suspiciously suspect. They always use "you" (the person they are asking the question of) or else some highly-esteemed figure such as Jesus ("What if Mary, a young unmarried mother, had chosen to abort..." as if, according to their own beliefs, God would somehow have chosen his "son" —

actually an alternative incarnation of himself — to be impregnated into someone who would make that choice) or Washington or Lincoln or Gandhi. They never seem to use as their examples those who actually were born to troubled, dysfunctional homes where they were unwanted, such as Adolf Hitler, Charles Manson or the street thug who broke into their home the week before.

Thought-questions on personhood:

a. Why are sperms and eggs not "human life" if they are alive and of the human species?

If "abortion is murder" ("killing" one insentient, preconscious "life"), then "menstruation is murder" (allowing one egg to die unfertilized) and "ejaculation is genocide" (killing hundreds of thousands of human lives).

b. In the case of **identical twins**, in the time after fertilization and the onset of cell division, but before the blastocyst actually divides into two entities, how many human persons exist? If only one, when did the second twin become a person if not at "conception"?

c. If cessation of brain waves is the standard for the end of life, how can you call it human life prior to the onset of EEG brain waves near the end of the 2nd trimester? Shouldn't the standard for the clinical *beginning* of life be the reciprocal of the standard for the clinical *end* of life?

d. Which would you save in a fire, a sleeping 3-year-old in her bedroom, or a frozen embryo in the freezer?

e. Let's say there are estranged brothers who are a good donor match. One needs the other to donate bone marrow to save his life, but the brother does not want to. They are both adults, undeniably human persons. Does one have the right to force another to use his body to keep him alive if the latter doesn't want to? They are both males. Does the requirement to use your body to keep someone else alive only apply to females?

f. Let's consider a purely hypothetical example to see if we are really willing to apply the same standards to men as to women. Let's imagine that the anti-choice extremists get their way and get conservative judges to repeal *Roe v. Wade* and outlaw abortion.

An unmarried couple, some time in a future conservative utopia, living in a state where abortion has been outlawed, has a one-night hookup and, a few weeks later, the woman informs the man that he is going to be a father. He implores her to get an abortion but, now illegal, she can't do that. She is forced by law to use her body to keep a pre-sentient fetus alive until birth. A week after birth, the infant is diagnosed with Leukemia and needs a bone marrow transplant. After checking available donors it is determined that only the child's *father* has a compatible match.

The father, who did not want the baby in the first place, says "NO!" ... IF you believe a woman should be forced to use her body to keep an embryo/fetus alive, do you also believe the state should also be able to compel the Father of the baby (with threats of fines and prison) to submit and have some of his bone marrow extracted to save his baby's life? Keep in mind that bone marrow, like its cousin the blood transfusion, is far less invasive or demanding of time than nine months of a pregnancy and, like a transfusion, is fully restored without permanent loss in a relatively short period of time.

At this point, we are no longer even dealing with the question of whether the offspring is a human person or not. This is no longer an embryo or a fetus that many believe a woman should be forced to use her body to sustain. It is now clearly a full-fledged, biologically autonomous sentient human baby.

Should a male parent be subject to the same demand that he be forced to use his body to keep his child — unambiguously a child, not a fetus — alive?

Even if he didn't want the pregnancy in the first place?

Even if he is estranged from the mother (and the baby, too)?

Even if he possibly has religious objections to any kind of transfusion?

Aside from the moral issue, should the state hold the father to the same standard as the mother?

Should any exception be allowed?

Qualitative Differences Between Human Persons and Other Life Forms

What is it about the essential nature of a human person that makes it *qualitatively different* than a rat, fish, insect, bacterium or virus? And by that I mean, why is a human person more special? Why is a human person inherently more valuable? What are the *qualities* of a human person that render intrinsic value that a rat or fish doesn't have?

I have stated that they are rooted in the *qualitative* distinctions that are unique to our species: conscious sentience and a capacity for reflective thought and self-examination, and the *actual* physical, emotional, mental and spiritual capabilities, features and processes that make such a distinction possible (as distinguished from the mere genetic blueprint or *potential* to develop those features).

One could say that the closer primitive creatures come to such abilities, the more intrinsic value or inherent worth they have — the closer they come to the *qualitative* values of human personhood, even if they are not actually human. Most people would be far more outraged by the wanton killing of a chimpanzee, gorilla, dolphin or whale than they would a rat or a fish or especially non-vertebrate life.

Why?

Clearly none of these animals is a human person. But they have many of the *qualitative* equivalents to a sufficient extent that we accord them much the same value. Even so, it has never been demonstrated that *any* of them, including chimpanzees, have the uniquely human attributes of moral self-examination, multi-generational historical perspectives or broad capabilities of abstract scientific or mathematical reasoning.

A human has human DNA and a rat has rat DNA. The DNA (deoxyribonucleic acid) is substantively different just because the arrangement of A's, T's, C's and G's of the genome sequencing (nucleotide base pairs of *adenine* [A] and *thymine* [T] or *cytosine* [C] and *guanine* [G] respectively) are different in an empirically observable and objectively quantifiable way. No problem. They are **quantitatively** identifyable according to their respective species. But why are they **qualitatively** different? Why does the label "human" make it intrinsically more valuable than the label "rat"?

A baby that has been born has *all* of the *actual* attributes of this kind of humanness, though they are very primitive at this early stage of development. But all of the physical features (a brain with measurable EEG brain waves, the supportive organs and bodily tools for operating on the environment) and emotional tools (the ability to express pain, anger, emotional and physical needs) and mental tools (the beginnings of actual cognitive interaction with its surrounding environment) actually exist. Again, they are new and young and just getting started, but they are all there.

But even if one says that a baby does not actually have all of these fully-functioning uniquely human capabilities (moral self-examination, historical perspectives, abstract reasoning), and perhaps has not attained full personhood, one does have to draw the line somewhere. Clearly NO first trimester zygote or embryo has *any* of these actual features or functions.

Clearly most human persons after a few years of life have all of them to some degree. And even damaged brains in comas or a persistent vegetative state DO maintain quite extensive repositories of actual personal experience as well as active EEG brain waves (the cessation of which allows the pronouncement of legal death), as well as the possibility of coming out of the coma.

So it appears reasonable that if many of the attributes of personhood don't even begin to fully manifest themselves in their full humanity until some time after birth (though the features and processes out of which they derive are fully extant at birth), and birth is the point at which the most private part of a woman's body is no longer being occupied, and care can possibly be transferred to others who are willing, then birth is a logical point at which to draw an absolute line on the beginning of personhood at which point the question of personhood can no longer be doubted.

Certainly if one really wants to play it conservatively, one could say that an absolute minimal standard would be the onset of EEG brain waves, which occurs at about 25 weeks pregnancy, near the middle of the second trimester, since even fishes and reptiles (vertebrates) have measurable EEG brain waves. So full personhood — full humanity — must commence at some point not merely *at* the onset of EEG brain waves, but some undefined point *after* that.

And as we have noted before, if the *end* of measurable EEG brain waves defines the end of personhood, certainly the time *before* that onset is a minimal standard for the onset of personhood.

Human Personhood and other issues

While not directly related to the issue of abortion, there are other contemporary issues that are influenced by considerations as to when a human *life* becomes a human *person* with its own individual rights.

Belief that there is no difference in the moral equivalence of living human tissue of a fetus, that has no measurable EEG brain waves, no feelings, no thoughts, no capacity for experience (though somehow failing to apply the same standard to the human lives of sperms and eggs), and an actual human person that has been born, is biologically autonomous, has feelings and has thoughts and experiences, creates a certain moral injustice. It means that, in the name of that fetal tissue's "rights," real human persons will be denied therapies and treatments that are already available now or which will be prevented from becoming available because the research is not permitted.

We can consider some of these issues in light of considering the difference between **human *life*** and **human *personhood***:

Embryonic Stem Cells (Research and therapies)

Immediately after a human egg cell is fertilized by a human sperm cell, when those who are most extreme believe a full human being with rights equal to yours (including the right to control your body), even though it has no feelings or thoughts about the subject, the single diploid cell, newly formed from the combination of two haploids, begins to divide. For a brief period of time, with each of the cell divisions, the new cells are exactly the same as each other. At that point, each cell is the same as every other cell in the organism, and each of those cells contains the DNA (deoxyribonucleic acid) coding such that it could grow into any part of a new human life's body.

At this point, the cells are extremely flexible, adaptable and versatile. Soon, as millions of new cell divisions lead to many more cells being created, they begin to specialize and begin developing into the specific body parts they will eventually become, based on where they are located in the growing physical body. They will then still hold the entire genetic blueprint, but their flexibility in being able to adapt to any environment and become any body part will be limited by the environment into which they have specialized into more clearly-defined roles.

Prior to settling into narrow, specific roles, these flexible, versatile, adaptable cells are known as "embryonic" stem cells. And science has learned that these cells hold enormous potential for healing damaged bodies and restoring body parts ravaged by illness or injury. Because these cells are so adaptable, they can be inserted into any damaged organ or body part, sense the environment they are in, adapt to it, and grow into new, young, healthy, undamaged tissue to replace that which is damaged ... *if* they are allowed to do so.

There are some who want to make sure they never get that chance.

Extremists who believe that a human person comes into existence at the moment a human egg is fertilized by a human sperm cell also believe that a one-celled, pre-specialization, pre-sentient organism has the moral equivalence of a fully-formed, biologically autonomous female adult, with an equal moral right to occupy and control her body.

This same line of "reasoning" also leads to the belief that this very early-stage, pre-specialization organism should not be created for any reason other than to be allowed to grow into a born human person. Thus, they consider any effort to create fertilized embryos and preserve them in a state of embryonic stem cells for the purposes of **research** or for therapeutic **treatments** to prevent or cure genetic disorders or to regenerate new tissue caused by injuries, illnesses (inherited or otherwise) or which have degenerated due to the normal processes of aging, to be the moral equivalent of murder. In contrast, most non-extremists see such research, treatments and therapies as miracles bestowed by science.

Research uses stem cells for experimentation to understand genetic science. This research and development leads to the production and administration of treatments for genetic disorders.

In order to research, experiment and develop the means for potential practical uses, embryos are produced, stored and used in research experiments. In the course of such experimentation, many cells are discarded and die, or are consumed in the process of utilizing them in objective, replicable studies.

Extremists who equate such cell tissue with sentient, autonomous human persons consider each

42

such use that causes individual fertilized embryos to be lost as the moral equivalent of murder.

Therapies actually implement the fruits of research. While research develops, discards and consumes fertilized embryonic cell tissue to develop potential practical uses, therapeutic implementation of those practical applications is what turns the potential human benefit into actual human benefit.

And, as with research, the process of actually producing, harvesting and utilizing embryonic cells, which some consider to be human persons representing the moral equivalent of human adults, also results in many going unused or being consumed in the process which, again, the extremists consider to be murder.

The mindset of such extremism is to claim that real human persons who need treatments to repair nerve cells, cure spinal cord injuries or regenerate lost or damaged body parts in the same way they were originally created in the embryonic environment, must be denied such reparative or restorative therapies because the "rights" of a pre-sentient, non-conscious, non-autonomous bit of cell tissue outweigh the rights of actual human persons who at least know they have them.

In Vitro Fertilization (IVF)

While in vitro fertilization is considered commonplace today and there is only limited objection, when it was first developed in the 1970's, it was opposed as vigorously and aggressively as stem cell research and therapies are today.

In vitro fertilization was ridiculed as creating "test tube babies" or "playing god" or creating "Franken-babies." (Funny how extremists so commonly ridicule any new life-saving medical advances as "playing god" until they or their loved ones are the ones being cured of illness, injury, pain or death or until such treatments become commonplace.)

The first baby actually produced through in vitro fertilization was Louise Brown, born July 25, 1978 in Oldham, England. As of this writing, she is a happy, productive adult woman, wife and mother. Millions of other babies have now been produced using the same treatments and, while there are still some of the most extreme who consider it to be the moral equivalent of murder because of the number of unused embryos that are discarded in the process, the controversy has largely subsided. Today, in vitro fertilization has blessed the lives of so many infertile or same-sex couples who would not otherwise have been able to conceive.

I would challenge anyone who still ridicules this important treatment option or mocks "test tube babies" or "Frankenbabies," to say that to the face of Louise Brown or as they look into the face of any new born miracle developed through this amazing, life-changing medical and scientific advance, which was made possible by standing up to the extremists by those not blinded by their superstition-driven ideological dogma.

Embryonic screening

Since the discovery of deoxyribonucleic acid (DNA) and advances in our ability to analyze, sequence and derive medical diagnosis and therapies based on DNA, new understanding and treatments have emerged.

In particular, the ability to identify the specific genetic combinations that result in birth defects or disabilities and test for their presence in the earliest stages of embryonic development, have led to the development of new tools for empowering parents in making medical and reproductive choices.

Some of the disabling conditions and genetic predispositions to disease that can now be identified in advance by genetic testing include Huntington's Disease, breast cancer likelihood identified by the BRCA1 gene, Tay-Sachs and many others. And the list keeps growing.

The problem for those who equate early-stage, pre-sentient human embryos with full-fledged human persons, is that the testing of embryos requires multiple embryos, and those with markers for disabling conditions or genetic predisposition to illness will likely be discarded. To anti-choice extremists, creating embryos with the knowledge and intent that some will be destroyed is the moral equivalent of murder.

To the rest of us, it is empowering families to reproduce with confidence that they are creating the best possible quality of life for themselves and the children they choose to bring into the world.

And again, noting that human eggs and human sperm are also human life, the same people who display such concern for the well-being of pre-sentient, early-stage embryos show very little regard for the well-being of those human eggs and sperms prior to fertilization.

Cloning (Reproductive or research or autologic therapies)

While embryonic stem cell research and therapies and in vitro fertilization have overcome initial early resistance to become largely favored by the general public, despite pockets of resistance among the most religiously conservative, and embryonic screening to test for genetic disabilities is rapidly moving in that direction, other opportunities for reproductive or research advances have not been so well-received as of the time of this writing.

It is possible, however, that just as embryonic stem cell research and therapies and in vitro fertilization have risen above their initial resistance to become widely accepted, that as some of these newer avenues of research and treatment come into more widespread awareness and implementation, that in time they will also find broader general acceptance.

The first of these is human cloning, for purposes of research, development of treatment using one's own newly-formed embryonic stem cells or, hypothetically, as yet another option in the areas of reproductive choice.

The first successful cloning of complete animals, first achieved successfully in mammals with Dolly the sheep, was announced on February 22, 1997, by Ian Wilmut, the lead researcher, along with Keith Campbell and colleagues at the Roslin Institute, part of the University of Edinburgh, Scotland.

The initial response by the public was revulsion and, like embryonic stem cell research and therapies and in vitro fertilization in their early days, invoked comparisons to "playing god" and "Frankenstein" monsters.

And this was towards a sheep, not a human being. Clearly, the implication was that if this could be done with sheep, it could (and would) soon be applied to humans.

While the emphasis was clearly on research and developing therapeutic treatment options, it was the mental image of producing exact genetic duplicates that captured the imagination of innovative thinkers and sparked the fears of those who found such ideas to be repulsive.

Yet even cloning for research and treatment was immediately opposed by religious extremists who equated cloning with, again, "playing god" and creating human embryos — human lives — with the intent that these lives would never live beyond that embryonic stage. Creating life knowing that it was never intended to live as its own separate organism, no matter what other scientific or treatment benefits might be gained, was seen as morally objectionable.

And while there has never been any serious pursuit of human cloning for reproduction, the idea did raise some interesting issues for conjecture.

First, it needs to be clarified that, despite references in popular culture, it is not the same as putting yourself into a human copying machine and getting an exact double of yourself. If a clone were to be produced, it would be a new little baby with the exact same genetic coding as yourself.

But that would be all. It would have the same genes, but not the same environment. It would grow up in a different generation, a different cultural milieu, be exposed to different family and social environments, different experiences and exposed to different foods and different environmental stimuli, both for better or worse. Newer immunization strategies might make this copy more protected against exposure to infectious illness, and greater environmental pollution might render it more vulnerable to increased environmental toxicity.

Again, some people found the idea of an exact genetic copy of a human being to be creepy. But that is really only because it was something new. It was not really so much the idea of a genetic duplicate that brought on the "yuck" factor, but more the idea that it was genetically engineered in the laboratory instead of the uterus. We know this because there does exist, as part of nature, exact genetic duplicates of humans.

They are known as identical twins. People are not repulsed by naturally occurring identical twins; they are fascinated by them! Many people fantasize about having a twin, or wish they could be a twin. So no, it is not the idea of a genetic duplicate that people find yucky, only the idea that it is something new and different and outside their comfort zone.

And further to the earlier point that a clone would not be an exact duplicate because it grows up in a different home environment, different generation and exposed to a different set of environmental and social stimuli, twins (the vast majority of whom are NOT "separated at birth" but who grow up together) usually do grow up in a very similar shared home life with very similar exposures to social, environmental and other shared stimuli, and yet they still are not exactly the same. They share the exact same genes, but despite many very fascinating similarities, they often develop those similarities in very different ways and, while some twins celebrate the sameness of their twinship, others seek to establish very different and unique individual personalities.

Another objection, less spoken of out loud, is that some men may object to the idea of genetic cloning because they threatened by the idea that women could be granted such reproductive autonomy as to render their role in the process unnecessary. Again, there is no basis for fear or concern. Like in vitro fertilization therapies, cloning would be an extremely invasive and expensive procedure, and not taken lightly. And human hormones and pheromones being what they are, and the social dance and romance of attraction and dating and mating, and all that leads to, the reality is that reproduction the good ol' fashioned way is not going anywhere soon, and no one needs to have any fear about anything.

But again, it must be emphasized that there are currently no proposals or the viable promise of human cloning for reproduction coming any time soon. In contrast, human cloning for research and the development of treatment options is already being advanced and is moving forward at a rapid pace, despite the many unfounded objections that remain.

And non-human cloning to rapidly produce bio-chemical materials used in treatments and research has been going on for many years and is well established and is the basis of many thriving genetic and biochemical industries in the fields of life science.

Birth Control

While the issue of a woman's right to use birth control is no longer as controversial as it was at other times in the past, when many states outlawed it altogether (before those laws were overturned by the case of *Griswold v. Connecticut* discussed at greater length in the chapter on legal issues), we need to remember that the acceptance of birth control, while widespread in our present era, is still not unanimous even today.

The Catholic Church in particular, as well as some other minor conservative religious denominations, continue to assert that artificial birth control, not being natural, is therefore contrary to the laws of God, and a violation of morality — notwithstanding that almost all Catholic women disregard this and practice birth control at some point in their lives.

This presents several ironies:

1. It undermines the credibility and control of an institution for which credibility and control are its lifeblood.

2. The Catholic Church owns and operates some of the leading research, scientific and medical facilities in the world, and is often at the forefront of bringing advanced medical care to those who might not otherwise be able to access it. Many of the medical technologies proudly embraced by the Catholic Church clearly prolong life in unnatural ways, and every surgical or medicinal intervention contravenes the course of nature as it would be if we left it entirely to God's hands. Most patients, even devout believers, and even if they are in a Catholic facility being attended to as closely by nuns as by surgeons, if given a choice between only surgery and only prayer (appealing purely to God and nature), would choose the surgery.

3. Many of the institutions that protest the loudest against birth control are also the ones who are even more vocal in their opposition to abortion. They fail to recognize the irony that the very birth control they oppose so loudly — a proactive, preventive measure — is the single most effective means of preventing the reactive, intrusive measure of terminating an unwanted pregnancy.

The Catholic prohibition against birth control was a modern response to an emerging technology, when artificial birth control by medication was developed and became widely available in the early 1960's.

Prior to that time, there were no scriptural, canonical or encyclical authorities on the subject because the technology was new and had not been previously addressed.

Many believe that if Pope John XXIII, a popular "people's pope" beloved much in his time as is Pope Francis at the time of this writing, had not died in 1963, less than five years after taking office, that he might have been more amenable to the real needs and feelings of real people, and might have ruled that such proactive medical treatments, not opposed by scripture or precedent, were permissible.

But following his untimely death, Pope John XXIII was succeeded by the more stern, legalistic Pope Paul VI who, in 1968, wrote the encyclical *Humanæ Vitæ* that pronounced artificial, medical birth control to be an unnatural interference with God's role in creating life.

Now that Pope Francis is at the head of the Catholic Church, and shaking things up, many suspect the possibility that Pope Paul VI's non-scriptural response to an emerging technology in his day, one that is now widely accepted and widely used even by Catholics, could possibly be reversed. Such a move would end one of the most widely flouted prohibitions in religious history, and put an end to the hypocrisy that is a key factor in undermining confidence in and obedience to the church.

We can only wait and see.

End of Life Options

At the opposite end of the same spectrum of life and personhood, is the flip side of the issue of abortion: end of life options.

Increasingly, those who wish to make their own choices about their lives are demanding the right to decide when the conditions of their lives become such that the quality of life is no longer worth continuing. They seek the right to determine that they should be able to terminate lives of pain and suffering.

As of the time of this writing, four U.S. states, beginning with Oregon in 1997, have enacted laws to permit physician-assisted suicide for patients with terminal illnesses who have less than six months to live. Carefully-worded safeguards protect against suicide for reasons of mental illness, pressure from heirs, lack of sound mind with insufficient capacity for valid consent or misdiagnosis of terminal conditions. Following Oregon in 1997, Washington, Montana and Vermont have enacted similar laws, and other states are currently considering similar options.

Many of the same institutions most vocal in their opposition to abortion (and often birth control) are the same ones who object to allowing those suffering painful deaths to make the voluntary choice to end their own suffering.

There are some people who do want to fight to the end. Others do not. Those who wish to fight or who wish to comply with the directives of religious advisors should have the full freedom to cling to life, no matter the consequences, for as long as they can.

Who gets to Choose?

They should have that right for themselves. They should **not** have the right to impose their choices and their beliefs on others who may feel differently.

Again: **Who gets to choose?**

Accepting Responsibility and Consequences

Returning to issues more directly related to the right to abort an unwanted pregnancy, some have argued that if one has consented to consensual sexual intimacy, one must accept the responsibility (consequences) for that decision, including the responsibility for possible pregnancy.

Consent to *sex* does not have to be consent to *pregnancy* any more than consent to riding in a car is consent to an automobile accident, even though both are possible secondary but unwanted, unintended and, in most cases, unlikely outcomes, although in both cases practicing safe, educated behaviors helps reduce the likelihood of accidents.

In any case, in the event of an automobile accident, accepting responsibility does not require that one be left to bleed to death at the scene of the accident. Medical remediation is sought to minimize physical and emotional trauma and to do everything possible to limit negative consequences. That is part of taking responsibility. In the same way, consequences of sexual intimacy may include medical intervention and, if the woman decides that abortion is part of the medical remediation that is right for her, then that can very well be an important aspect of accepting responsibility.

This whole line of argument demonstrates the intent to impose one's personal moral or religious opinions onto others who may not hold the same beliefs.

Even a completely voluntary sex act would not necessarily mean she invited the embryo into her body, since only a small percentage of sex acts result in pregnancy. The *possibility* of an outcome is very different than its *intent*. If a person rides in a car, knowing there is the *possibility* of an accident, should that person be denied the right to receive medical care, auto repairs or reimbursement from a responsible party if they have an accident ... since they *knew* that was a *possible* outcome? A woman who has sex only invites the sharing of sexual intimacy, not the embryo that accidentally resulted. And **even if** she got pregnant on purpose, there is no reason to say that a person can't change their mind or correct a mistake, especially when it is the rights of an actual human person against those of non-sentient cell tissue with the potential of becoming a person ... if the woman wants it.

Suppose I invite someone over for a drink. He stays and stays. He becomes obnoxious, in fact. I decide I don't like him and regret having invited him to come inside in the first place. I want him gone. I have as great a right to evict him as I would if he were a burglar. The fact that I previously thought I wanted him there (or I simply change my mind) does not make me lose the right to control who stays in my house. And a woman's body is far more personal and intimate than a structure of wood and stucco.

When a man forcibly enters and occupies the most private, personal, intimate part of a woman's reproductive anatomy against her will, we call it "rape." Though it only lasts for a few moments (barring additional physical assault and injury), the trauma and emotional scars can last for years. Yet there are some who would require, by force of law, that women be mandated to have that most private part of their bodies occupied by an unwanted intruder for nine long months. The trauma and emotional scars of a forced, unwanted pregnancy can harm a woman just as long as a rape, and also traumatize the child that is born unwanted.

In any case this argument automatically validates abortion in the case of rape or incest where there was no such consent at all. No person who raises an argument against abortion based on consent to sex can possibly raise an objection in cases where such consent did not exist.

The questions of when human life begins, when human life becomes a human person and questions that weight the "rights" of pre-sentient cell tissue against the rights of fully conscious, fully sentient human persons — the question, in the case of each issue of **who gets to choose** — are at the core of the issue of a woman's right to abort an unwanted pregnancy.

But as we have seen in this chapter, abortion is not the only issue affected by such questions. And in the clash of moral philosophies, and how public policies should be brought to bear — by force of law

— on the full spectrum of such issues and choices, we consistently see that those who claim to equate human **life** with human **personhood**, despite their inconsistency in omitting the human life of human sperm and egg cells, remain dogmatic in their intent to impose their beliefs and values on those who feel differently.

Those who support the right of a woman to choose to terminate an unwanted pregnancy, or a terminally ill person to choose to end their suffering, or scientific advances that can cure diseases, or expanded options for new technologies to assist those who choose to be pregnant but wrestle with fertility issues, all respect the right of any person who holds different views to put those beliefs into practice *in their own lives.*

But we adamantly reject the notion that they have the right to impose those beliefs on others.

Who gets to choose?

2

LEGAL ASPECTS OF
REPRODUCTIVE RIGHTS

We have clearly established in Chapter One that a human blastocyst / zygote / embryo / fetus is alive — ergo, "human life," but that it is not a human person, any more than a human sperm or egg cell, also human life long before fertilization.

On that basis alone, if there is no moral basis for equating the "rights" of a *potential* human person with those of the *actual* person who owns the body being occupied, there can be no valid moral basis at all on which to claim that it should be unlawful for a woman to terminate a pregnancy that she does not wish to continue.

A being, even if a life, that has no feelings, no consciousness, no sentience nor even the awareness of its own existence, much less any sense of "rights" or justice. "Rights" emanate from the capacity of a being to exercise free will and to experience the consequences of its choices. A life form that does not even have the capacity for experiencing "rights" has no capability or basis for such "rights" to even exist.

Even so, for those who do not accept the conclusions in Chapter One about the differentiation between human life and being a human person, one can hold the opinion that human personhood begins at fertilization and still recognize the moral basis for allowing a woman the legal right not to have her body used to keep someone else alive if she does not wish to do so willingly.

Abortion in United States Law — past and present

Since January 1973, the supreme judicial standard governing abortion in the United States, by order of the United States Supreme Court, has been the case of *Roe v. Wade* (410 U.S. 113 [1973]).

Opposition to the case of *Roe v. Wade* has often been expressed as objecting to a "liberal" court "legislating from the bench" to overturn long-standing traditional values that have always been respected in the past, going back to the time of Founders who wrote the Constitution.

The anti-choice conservatives are convinced that the Founders would be outraged — turning over in their graves — that such a decision could claim a constitutional basis.

Those taking this view demonstrate a lack of familiarity with this case or with the "tradition" of reproductive law in the history of the United States.

The decision in *Roe v. Wade* was not a close decision. It was decided 7-2, with the decision written by Harry Blackmun, a moderately conservative Republican appointed to the Supreme Court by President Richard M. Nixon.

The decision was based on respect for tradition, respect for personal liberty and free choice, and interpreting the Bill of Rights according to the *intent of the Founders* who had actually written the Constitution.

Here are the historical facts about abortion in United States history: at the time this nation was founded, abortion up until the perception of fetal movement ("quickening"), which usually occurs near the beginning of the second trimester, *was fully legal in all thirteen colonies* that became the thirteen original states.

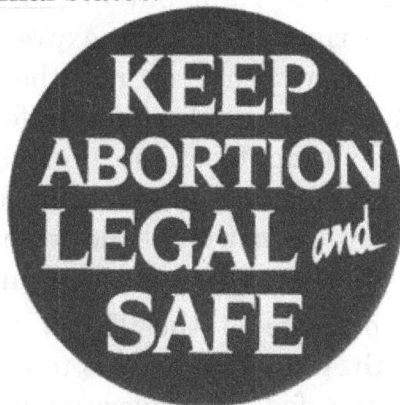

Under governing English Common Law, there were *no laws against first trimester abortion any-*

61

where in the thirteen original colonies, and this
continued after the thirteen colonies became the
thirteen States. Further, Common Law also mandated that, even in the case of illegal abortions (after
"quickening"), the woman herself was immune from
prosecution.

This point is explicitly discussed in *Roe v. Wade* at
great length, in Section VI.3-5 of the decision, to
demonstrate that when the Founders referred to
being secure in one's home or person, their mindset
would include the right of a woman to be safe from
intrusive government oppression in dictating control
of the most private part of her body.

The Court had previously taken the standard of
having imputed a "penumbra" right of privacy in the
earlier case of *Griswold v. Connecticut* (381 U.S. 479
[1965]) regarding contraceptive rights. Like a
number of other states, Connecticut had outlawed
not only abortion, but also even birth control. But in
Roe, the Court came right out and said there is a
direct, absolute right of privacy expressly stated in
the Constitution, whether or not the actual word
"privacy" is there, just as the many references in the
Constitution to voting, elections, etc., create a clear,
specific and unambiguous intent to have a represen-
tative democracy, even though no form of the word
"democracy" occurs anywhere in the Constitution.

The whole premise of the Third, Fourth, Fifth,
Sixth and Ninth Amendments was to protect privacy
from acts of the federal government, which was
extended to protection from acts of state govern-

ments via the incorporation doctrine established by the Fourteenth Amendment.

As to the intent of the Founders based on law and custom, abortion was legal in all colonies that became states, and remained so for almost fifty years after becoming independent from Great Britain.

The first state to actually pass a law outlawing abortion was Connecticut, in 1821 (32 years after passage of the Bill of Rights; 45 years after the Declaration of Independence), followed by New York (1828), with a law that was subsequently modeled by many other states. By the end of the 19th century, abortion had been outlawed in all states.

By the mid 1960's, opinions had begun to change in the United States, and some states began to restore the legal status that had existed at the time of the Founders.

Prior to *Roe,* 16 states comprising almost half the population of the United States had already legalized abortion, including the large population centers of New York and California, whose statute legalizing abortion, the California Therapeutic Abortion Act, was signed into law by then-governor Ronald Reagan as one of his first acts, early in the first of his two terms as California governor.

Abortion deaths and legal status: In 1966, when abortion was illegal in all states, on the cusp of a revolution to reverse that, there were 120 deaths from abortion. In 1972, just before *Roe v. Wade,* when abortion was legal in 16 states with significant populations, abortion deaths dropped to 39.

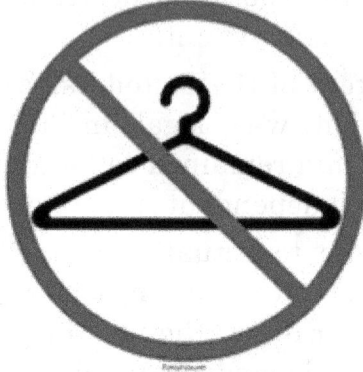

By the 1980's, after Roe, with abortion legal (if not always accessible) in all states, abortion deaths dropped to 10-20 per year. Clearly, legalizing women's rights to make their own medical choices about their own bodies has led to saving women's lives.

Bodily Sovereignty

Personal choices about behavior should never be legislated, unless and until they infringe the equal rights of other persons. The old saying goes, "Your right to swing your fist ends where my nose begins."

Persons have the right to make any choices they want about their behavior, including moral choices, up to the point that they infringe someone else's equal rights.

A person has the right to wear whatever they want, choose the color of their house, or even choose to engage in sexual behavior (alone or with others who have the capacity to consent to free and voluntary participation) and, however much someone else may disapprove of their taste or moral beliefs, they have the right to make those choices as long as they do not cause harm to others or infringe other persons' rights to the equal moral or aesthetic choices *they* believe to be appropriate.

Rights of the Woman vs. Rights of Embryo

The problem in the case of abortion is that the disagreement about abortion is partially about differing moral beliefs, but also a disagreement about whose rights are being infringed. Those opposed to abortion claim that they are protecting the rights of the zygote/embryo/fetus from the infringement of having its life terminated.

But even if the zygote/embryo/fetus were a fully-endowed human person, with all the rights of personhood, all the way back to the moment of fertilization, the crux of the *legal* question becomes, "Who has the right to control the body: the zygote/embryo/fetus occupying it or the woman who owns it?"

Who gets to choose?

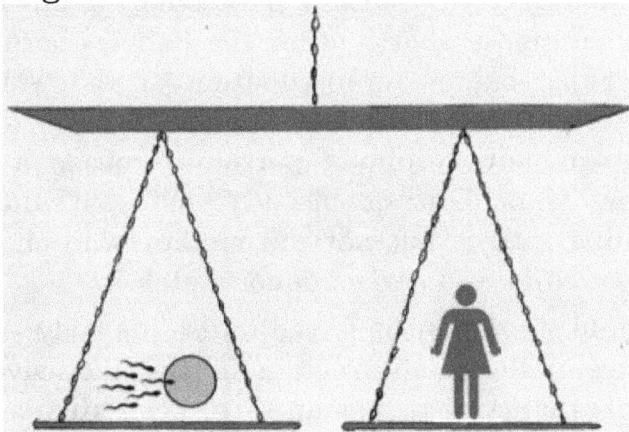

Who Owns the Body?

Who owns a body? Who has a right to make decisions about life based on that body?

At this point, perhaps we ought to revisit a couple of the thought-questions from Chapter One (Life vs. Personhood), but adapt them from the question of personhood to the question of whether other people are held to the same standard of being required by law to use their bodies to keep someone else alive:

Should an identical twin be required by force of law to donate an organ to his estranged brother, a perfect genetic match, to keep him alive? How about something less intrusive than an organ: how about bone marrow or a blood transfusion? No one would question that it is morally desirable for the brother to come to the aid of his twin, but what if he doesn't want to? Should he be forced to use his body to keep his estranged brother alive?

How about an unwed father who wanted his pregnant girlfriend to get an abortion and, when she did not agree, was forced to become an unwanted father? Suppose shortly after the baby is born, and neither personhood or occupation of the woman's body continues to be the issue, the baby — who is unambiguously a human person — needs a bone marrow transplant or blood transfusion and the unwilling father, but not the mother who chose to bear the child, is a perfect donor match.

Should the father be forced to use his body — at a infinitesimally small fraction of the intrusiveness that pregnancy is to woman — to keep alive a baby he did not want if he does not agree to do so?

Should men — identical but estranged twin brothers or unwilling fathers — be held to the same legal standard as women in requiring, by force of law, that they use their bodies to keep others alive?

[The full scenarios are examined in more depth in the section "thought-questions on personhood" in Chapter One.]

Good Samaritan Laws

While most people consider it a praiseworthy act to help out a stranger, nowhere in any jurisdiction within the United States is there a legal mandate that one must help someone in need, and this is also the standard in most nations around the world.

Over the decades, there have been occasional proposals to require people to come to the aid of strangers if the need is serious and if the inconvenience to the would-be "Good Samaritan" would be minimal. But none of these laws has ever actually been enacted, partly because it is difficult to objectively define a standard of seriousness in operational terms that would clearly spell out when it would rise to the level of imposing an obligation on those around, who would be required to provide such services (i.e., would a medical doctor be required to come forward and offer medical aid in ways that other people would not? what about a registered nurse? a licensed vocational nurse?), or what level of inconvenience would be tolerable to justify the imposition of a positive duty to take action that is backed up by force of law?

If a person of means sees a hungry person starving on the street, would they have a legal obligation to buy them a meal if it would not pose a significant level of inconvenience? How many starving people would they have to provide for before it became an inconvenience? What level of income would earn the right to be subject to that imposition?

What about if you see someone drowning? Would you be required by law to try to save them? What if you can't swim? What if you are on your way to the airport for a non-refundable flight for your daughter's wedding?

How do you define the standard for requiring someone else to provide aid? How do you define what constitutes a reasonable level of inconvenience?

Pregnancy and motherhood can be noble conditions that bring joy to many. But not every woman finds every pregnancy convenient, wanted or joyful.

While one might find admiration for a woman who chooses to endure an unwanted pregnancy and bear a child for someone else to adopt, how do you define a standard of inconvenience that can or should be imposed by force of law?

To be or not to be a hero: Who gets to choose?

Is Abortion Murder?

Not all killing is murder.

Killing for lawful execution is not murder.

Killing as part of war is not murder.

Killing in self-defense is not murder.

68

Killing that is not against the law is not murder.

Killing of something that is **not a person** is not murder.

Killing a bacterium is not murder.

Killing more complex non-human life, such as an insect or animal pest or even meat for food is not murder.

Killing a **human life** that is not a human person, such as an unfertilized egg or sperm — or a newly-fertilized embryo or zygote — is not murder.

Is Meat Murder?

While I am fully "pro-choice" on the subject of eating meat, it must be noted that vegetarians could absolutely make a stronger case that "meat is murder" than the case anti-choice extremists could make that "abortion is murder."

Meat requires the killing of a sentient, autonomous animal that is **not** occupying the most private part of a human's body, and which is wholly unnecessary since humans can get all needed nutrients from plant sources such as fruits, nuts and vegetables that produce food without killing a sentient creature and, in many cases such as fruits, nuts many grains (depending on how they are harvested) or other vegetables, not even killing the plant! (Not only that, but consumptions of fruits and nuts by humans or other animals actually assists the plants in reproduction by helping to spread their seeds.)

In contrast, artery-clogging animal fat is wholly unnecessary to a healthy diet.

The definition of "murder" (as distinguished form mere "killing") has comprised the following three elements throughout time, including the time of the Hebrew lawgivers and other early contemporary civilizations whose primitive legal codes influenced the development of Western jurisprudence:

a) Intent — killing of a person is deliberate rather than accidental.

b) Malice or wantonness (i.e., not merely for defensive reasons or reasons of domestic or international law and order). Many would argue that the choice to terminate an unwanted pregnancy is self-defense of the most private part of a woman's body.

c) Killing of a **person** (not a virus, bacteria, insect, animal or human tissue that is alive but which is not a person, *i.e.,* sperm, egg, zygote, embryo, fetus).

A woman's intentional choice to terminate a pregnancy in the interest of her bodily sovereignty incorporates, at most, only the first of those elements; and, if the tissue removed is not even a human person or no moral issue is involved, then even that does not apply.

Legal Aspects of Abortion Funding

Aside from the issue of whether or not abortion should be legal as a matter of public policy, for the present time it is settled law that women have a Constitutional right of privacy and personal liberty to control their own bodies and choose whether or not they wish to continue with an unwanted pregnancy.

So the next question becomes, who should pay for abortions? Who should be financially responsible for ensuring access to a Constitutional right?

As of this writing, it is against the law in the United States to use federal money to pay for abortions. The Hyde Amendment was passed on September 30, 1976.

This law was introduced by Henry Hyde, a rabid anti-abortion extremist congressman and self-proclaimed moral arbiter from Illinois. This was the same Congressman Hyde who was one of the Congressional leaders and judgmental moralists who brought impeachment charges against President Bill Clinton on moral grounds, and was subsequently forced to step down when he himself was caught in adultery. The moral hypocrisy and double standard astounds.

Certainly, we don't expect public funding to ensure all rights. We have the right to freedom of speech, but we don't expect the government to buy us a printing press or television station. We have the right to freedom of religion, but governments do not pay for churches, though they do allow churches to operate as tax-deductible non-profit charities, even when they indisputably rake in huge profits and are led by megabillionaire pastors living in opulent, tax-free "parsonages."

Abortion is a medical procedure. As such, it does allow a tax deduction for medical expenses if one itemizes deductions rather than taking a standard

71

deduction, and if one's overall medical expenses are a sufficient percentage of one's income to qualify.

But beyond that, if a woman has a Constitutional right to this specific medical procedure, I would argue that it should be handled, at a minimum, the same as any other medical treatment under the law.

And while there are many who object on ideological grounds to any public funding of any health care access, the fact is that, in our present system, there are many instances in which there is funding for medical procedures.

We have Medicare for those over a certain age, which also includes younger people who qualify based on disability or income levels, which could include women of child bearing age; we have government employees who are covered for medical care under the terms of their employment; we have the Veterans Administration covering medical expenses for qualified military veterans and their families and more recently, with the enactment of the Affordable Care Act (often called "Obamacare"), we have public subsidies for medical coverage in state and federal health care marketplace exchanges.

Under these various programs, coverage is provided to **men** for reproductive care such as vasectomies and prescriptions for medications such as Viagra or Cialis to address issues of erectile dysfunction.

I certainly do not begrudge men the right to a full spectrum of coverage for their medical needs, including reproductive care. But I would absolutely argue for the equal right of women to have full and complete coverage for the entire spectrum of women's reproductive care, including prenatal care for wanted pregnancies, and abortions to terminate those that are not wanted.

There are no other instances in which one single segment of the population is singled out for denial of equal access to medical care, where corresponding equivalent care is provided to other groups, and especially for a specific medical procedure that the United States Supreme Court has defined as a Constitutional right.

It seems that the same Court that declared abortion a Constitutional right would recognize this but, sadly, as judicial appointments have changed the makeup of the Court, judicial ideologies are shifted and, while some justices may be unwilling to overturn an established precedent, even if they might have voted differently in the original underlying case, in honor of the judicial principle of *stare decisis* (honoring precedent) which affords stability and predictability to judicial proceedings, they might be willing to rein in the effects of the precedent by limiting the scope of its applicability. They may allow *Roe v. Wade* to stand, but limit the access to those who need the financial assistance of public funding, creating a two-tiered system of access — one standard for those of means and a lesser standard for those less fortunate — to what is supposed to be a Constitutional right enjoyed equally by everyone.

Limiting Availability of Clinics

In addition to trying to limit women's access to their right to terminate an unwanted pregnancy by the increasingly successful tactic of denying funding to those who need it most, another strategy is to limit the availability of local clinics.

Women who are financially comfortable who find themselves with an unwanted pregnancy always have the option of traveling to a place where there is easy access. Women who are financially challenged may not have such options.

Increasingly, we have seen states with conservative legislatures or judicial systems (or both) pass highly intrusive laws with restrictions on clinics that are only applied to facilities if abortions are performed. They include such things as requiring full operating rooms for a minor, in-office procedure, on-staff physicians with admitting privileges at local hospitals in areas where no hospital will admit physicians who perform abortions, which effectively prevents the clinic from operating, and other very extensive specifications for construction and access that do not apply to any other clinics.

The idea, of course, is to create a framework of regulatory complexity that is essentially impossible to comply with. So much for getting big, intrusive government off our backs. And since the regulations are designate as being applicable *only* to clinics where abortions are performed, the practical effect is to make abortion functionally illegal, without actually passing laws to prohibit it.

While no one would dispute that we need appropriate regulatory oversight of medical facilities to protect the health and safety of patients and the safe access to quality medical care by qualified physicians, when laws or regulations are enacted that only apply to one specific procedure — one that the Supreme Court has declared to be a Constitutional right — that is clearly singled out for ideological reasons, then validity of such laws and regulations must be challenged.

And in some jurisdictions, the opposite occurs: a liberal state legislature may enact laws to ensure access for abortion patients that the more conservative Supreme Court may overrule or restrict.

A recent example was the case of *McCullen v. Coakley* 573 U.S. _ (2014), in which the state of Massachusetts passed a law requiring a buffer zone of thirty-five feet around clinics providing abortions, keeping protesters away from clinic doors by at least that distance, to protect the privacy of abortion patients and to prevent them from being harassed and possibly assaulted by extremist protesters.

In that case, in which the liberal judges wrote separate concurrences to the majority opinion by Chief Justice John Roberts, the court issued a unanimous ruling that the protesters had a First Amendment free-speech right of protest and that the thirty-five foot buffer zone effectively infringed that right, and the Massachusetts law was overturned. The Court did, however, leave open the possibility that a shorter distance buffer zone might be permissible to protect a more immediate zone of privacy and

75

safety around patients. But with unsettling vagueness, the Court stopped short of specifying exactly where they would draw the line, thus inviting a return to this issue again at some future date.

Clearly, the judicial record is mixed.

In many cases, even in an era of increasingly conservative judicial rulings, courts have ruled laws restricting clinic access to be unconstitutionally void. But, as we have seen, the record is mixed, and many conservative legislatures continue to try to push the boundaries and test the courts to see just how far they can go in limiting access.

And the United States Supreme Court continues to be unpredictable in issuing mixed rulings as to which local and state laws and which lower court rulings they will allow to stand. And so, until the ideological balance on the Court shifts from several solid liberals and several solid conservatives, with a couple of swing votes in the middle, it seems that for the foreseeable future the judicial aspects of how women's reproductive care is decided will continue to be volatile.

Laws Requiring Parental Notification and Consent

Another tactic used by those seeking to restrict access to abortion without outlawing it altogether includes enacting laws requiring parental notification: requiring that parents or legal guardians be notified and, in some cases, consent to, the choice to terminate an unwanted pregnancy.

A girl who is old enough to be pregnant is old enough to make certain decisions that affect the rest of *her* life and which *she* more than anyone else will bear consequences for the rest of her life.

I have never seen a "parental notification" proposal that includes a requirement that the parents who make a decision opposite of what the girl wants be required to assume lifetime liability for responsibility and support of the child brought into the world by their decision. Nor do I hear anti-choice extremists talk much about the reciprocal of that situation: how would anti-choice conservatives feel about parents who think an abortion would be the best solution to a problem situation, but a defiant underage girl wants to carry her pregnancy to term? Would the conservatives also agree that the parents should have the right to impose mandatory abortion in cases where they do not consent to their daughter's pregnancy?

We are not talking about headaches and aspirin here, but life-changing consequences. An underage girl may not be old enough to make all adult decisions, or to consent to legal adult choices or even adult relationships, but if she is pregnant, whether she aborts, carries or gives the child up for adoption, *she* will be the one who endures the consequences for the rest of her life.

That is true whether she was forcibly raped, the victim of incest or "thought" she was in love and was trying to act like the adult that she isn't.

In any case, the examples of incest and child abuse are, alone, valid reasons why notification laws are not workable. Almost all girls with a problem situation will turn first to their parents for help. If a girl can't go to her parents with this kind of problem, then she should not have to.

And the alternative is ... what? A scared teenaged girl being forced to go to a judge? Give me a break! The whole point is to set up one more roadblock to make abortion harder. Newsflash! One of the key reasons for making abortion LEGAL is so she doesn't have to have a "do it yourself" or back-alley job. She IS going to be talking to adult professionals, even in the extremely rare instances in which she can't go to her parents.

Look at the reality: This issue is not about parental control. If she can't go to her parents with this kind of problem at this age, they have already lost control. This is about strangers forcibly stopping girls from having abortions at all.

This issue is further discussed in the chapter on additional issues in reproductive choice.

The bottom line is that, having previously established in Chapter One that there is no moral basis for considering a non-sentient, pre-conscious human life with the *potential* of becoming a fully-human *person,* to be the moral equivalent of an actual human person, there is also no moral basis for prohibiting abortion as a legal mandate, with that prohibition enforced by force of law.

Beyond that, even if that premise is rejected despite the overwhelming evidence to support it, even if the non-sentient, pre-conscious human life were fully human, there is no legal basis for mandating that one person be forced to use their body to keep another person alive if she does not voluntarily consent to do so, also recognizing the distinction between consent to sex and consent to pregnancy as one possible consequence of sexual intimacy.

There is no valid moral nor legal basis for prohibitions against a woman's right to make deeply personal choices about her own life and her own reproductive options.

3

ᕼBORTION
ᕼND JUᗡEO-CᕼRISTIᕼN RELIGION

ester Prynne, in Nathaniel Hawthorne's
Scarlet Letter, was subject to cruel punishment by public officials who used a grotesque
distortion of the religion they claimed is
based on a messianic "savior" who had reportedly
rebuked those trying to stone the adulteress.

So also, much of the thrust to dictate control over
the most private parts of women's bodies claims to
originate from Biblical teachings by those who have
no idea what the Bible actually does or does not say
about abortion, and who are quick to misrepresent
and distort the words and message of a book they
claim to accept as divine and inerrant.

It should first be pointed out that the Bible is a text of personal, private religious belief, not of public policy or law.

Some people believe the Bible to be the word of God; many others do not. Some believe in other scriptural authorities many do not believe in religion of any kind. In a secular nation of many faiths and traditions, no single system of beliefs or doctrines should be used as the basis for public policies or laws that affect everyone, nor should private religion ever be the basis for public policy.

With every bit the same level of hypocrisy as those who humiliated the young Puritan adulteress that Jesus would have forgiven, today's Puritans fail to understand that there is not a single word in the Bible against abortion. The Bible is completely pro-choice. Those who claim otherwise need to take their Bibles off their pedestals, blow off the dust, actually open them up for once and actually read what is in it, and this chapter will assist them in their search, including specific responses to the specific Bible verses the anti-choice extremists love to toss around.

The Bible is Pro Choice

While, again, whatever the Bible does or does not say about abortion should not be relevant to public policy issues, because so many people *do* believe in the Bible to be the inerrant and infallible word of their god, and cite it (in error) as their basis for opposing women's rights of reproductive self determination, this section is presented to address the concerns and questions of those whose religious tradition does include belief in the Bible and who let that influence their views on women's reproductive freedom.

Why are some conservative Christians, who claim the Bible as their sole moral authority, so opposed to abortion?

While abortion was well known and written about in ancient Hebrew times (some in favor, some against), *the **Bible** itself is completely silent on the subject of abortion.*

None of the other writings from that era, either supporting or opposing abortion, including those cited by those opposed to abortion, made it into the Bible, and citing such sources only reiterates that abortion *was* known to those in Bible times, yet still unmentioned by the Bible writers.

No specific passage in the Bible either encourages or discourages abortion.

The general silence about abortion is the way it should be: don't go to either extreme, to mandate forced pregnancy (like the religious extremists) or mandate forced abortion (like the Communists in China on the extreme left). The common denominator in tyranny from either the right (prohibiting abortion) or left (mandating it) is coercion by force of law.

In contrast, those who are pro-*choice,* respecting the woman's *right to choose* whether or not to be pregnant, want to get Big Theology, just like Big Intrusive government, off our backs and out of our bedrooms. Abortion is a matter should be left to each individual to decide in her own situation.

And the Bible agrees with this view.

The true Biblical view of abortion is *pro-choice*.

There *are* passages in the Bible that speak of birth, conception, accidental miscarriage, pregnancy, and the formation and creation of life, which are often cited as supporting the "sanctity of life" by those who can't find any actual reference to abortion.

Further, the Bible contains extremely detailed descriptions of what constitutes murder as well as what constitutes lawful and justifiable homicide. In fact, the Bible has many instances in which the "sanctity of life" is secondary to other considerations.

Any one of these subjects would have been a *perfect opportunity* for the Bible writers to include the simple statement that abortion is a sin, or is forbidden, or is murder, or whatever. **But they didn't.**

Religious extremists who claim that their only authority is a literal interpretation of the Bible, but who are against a woman's right to reproductive choice, are ignorant about religion as well as history. They have staked their message on the "Big Lie." The Bible is completely pro-choice.

Abortion in Bible Times

Abortion was well known and widely practiced in ancient times, during Old Testament domination by the Israelites as well as under the Roman domination at the time Jesus lived, as it has been in even the most primitive societies.

The Old and New Testaments are very outspoken on even very minute aspects of daily life, especially the Law of Moses. Jesus later clarified many of these laws to remove ambiguity or to add motive and intent to the spirit of the law.

If the commandments against murder were intended to apply to fetuses, then the Law of Moses, the later prophets and judges would have said so.

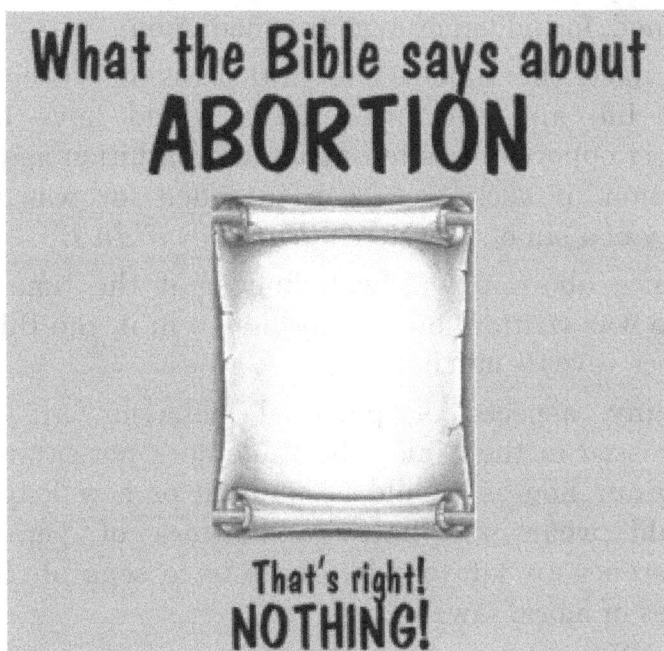

What the Bible says about
ABORTION

That's right!
NOTHING!

Or, if there were some misunderstanding or confusion about the subject, later prophets, or Jesus himself speaking hundreds of years later, could have provided some clarification on the subject.

At the very least, an omnipotent and omniscient God should have been able to foresee the future conflict in our time and just come right out and unambiguously state that commandments against killing were also applicable to abortion. *But they didn't.*

Yet, while the Law of Moses outlines penalties and conditions for various types of killing (neighbors, foreigners, intentional, etc.), along with various types of permissible and forbidden killing (self-defense, executions, wartime vs. homicides), there is not a single place in the Bible where abortion is condemned, forbidden or even frowned upon.

In fact, the Bible on several occasions discusses fetal life and existence. These would have been perfect opportunities to include a prohibition against abortion, if such had been intended (or was God guilty of a sin of omission?). *But they didn't.*

Since abortion was well known at the time the Bible was written, but not forbidden in it, the Bible's silence reveals much.

Many aspects of personal behavior are not addressed in the Bible. The Bible does not say what color our houses should be painted or how long we should wear our hair — matters of personal preference are left to individual *choice,* separate from issues of moral law.

In like manner, the Bible also does not encourage, support or promote abortion. It is neither pro-abortion nor anti-abortion. As with most other matters of personal prerogative, the Bible takes a neutral (silent) position, leaving the matter to individual discretion, or *choice.*

It may be the right choice for some individuals in some situations, and the wrong choice for others.

Since the scriptures are completely silent on the issue, they obviously intended this to be left to individual preference (i.e. *choice*). Those who claim Biblical authority to justify their human interpretations about a subject on which the Bible is silent are dishonest and hypocritical, or are listening to the misleading guidance of those who deliberately play on their beliefs to mislead them and exert control over their personal lives.

It is amazing that the Biblical authority is claimed for so many subjects where the Bible is actually silent or ambiguous (or even contradictory), while they completely ignore other parts of the Bible such as archaic commands in the Law of Moses (in the Biblical books of Exodus, Leviticus and Deuteronomy) in which the Bible is very clear, such as prohibiting tattoos or the eating of shrimp, pork or ham or demanding animal sacrifice or many aspects of religious observance and practice that seem prohibitively intrusive today. Yet today these inconvenient commandments that actually *are* in the Bible simply ignored by all but the most orthodox, while the same people who ignore what is actually in the Bible claim biblical authority in matters where the Bible is completely silent.

The religious conservatives deny obvious contradictions and they ignore specific commands that actually *are* in the Bible, and yet they claim Biblical authority on a subject *not in the Bible!*

So now let us take a look at some of what the Bible actually *does* say...

Specific Scriptures

The religious conservatives will usually admit a lack of any explicit prohibition of abortion of the Bible, but will cite various specific passages to imply an *intent* to oppose abortion. Following are a number of specific scriptural references that are often cited in a desperate attempt to try and claim a non-existent Biblical opposition to abortion.

While I have responded to each of these commonly-cited verses, it is important to note one key fact that they all have in common: they discuss birth, death, life, creation, pregnancy and pre-natal formation of the *body,* any of which would have been a perfect place to simply insert a clear an unambiguous statement opposing abortion (which was known and practiced in Bible times), but not one of these verses makes any reference whatsoever to either the existence of pre-natal ensoulment nor to even the slightest claim that abortion is the teensiest bit wrong.

Jeremiah 1:5: "Before I formed thee in the belly I knew thee; and before thou camest forth out of the womb I sanctified thee, [and] I ordained thee a prophet unto the nations." (KJV)

This scripture has traditionally been used by Protestants to show god's foreknowledge of long future events, and by Mormons to claim a pre-mortal existence of life in heaven prior to birth.

Only recently, since the move to re-legalize abortion beginning in the mid-twentieth century, have very desperate anti-choice extremists reinterpreted this in the context of abortion.

Look at the wording of this scripture, "Before I formed you in the womb...." It is talking about before birth, before viability ... *before conception!* Is that referring to sperms and eggs?

It has no relevance to abortion whatsoever; but if it shows reverence to *potential* life, it actually applies as much to sperms and eggs as to embryos, since it is prior to conception.

And even if it were a reference to embryonic life (it isn't), and no one denies the existence of embryonic life with the potential to become a human being and, once again, it would have been a perfect opportunity to condemn abortion, ***but didn't.***

In context, the passage is near the very beginning of the first chapter of the book of Jeremiah.

Jeremiah is introducing his ministry, and is writing in this first chapter specifically about his own calling as a prophet — that it was known by god before he was born or even conceived.

He was appointed, chosen, selected, ordained — whatever. He is talking about the fact that God knew of his calling long before he existed as a real or potential human.

Prior to *Roe v. Wade,* most Bible scholars interpreted this as a reference to God's foreknowledge of the future, and not until recently did the scripture ever enter into the abortion debates.

If anything, this reference to God's foreknowledge of the future suggests that He should have been able to foresee the modern controversy about abortion and taken the simple step of simply coming right out and said that it was wrong or prohibited, if he had any such intent. *But he didn't.*

Psalm 127:3: "Truly children are a *gift* from the *Lord;* the fruit of the womb is a reward." (KJV) As a parent and grandparent, I certainly agree!

But ... my daughter and granddaughters were the results of *wanted,* intentional pregnancies. Children are a gift, but the Bible writer certainly passed up a particularly ideal verse in which to universalize that concept, didn't he?

And we should remember the nature of a "gift" — a gift is freely given, and the recipient has the *option* (read: **choice**) to accept or reject the gift.

According to Judeo-Christian religious teaching, God gave us many "gifts." He created *everything,* and when he was done, he pronounced it "good." He also created viruses and bacteria and insects and mice. Do you ever feel "put upon" by these "gifts" and use injections or inoculations or bug spray or mousetraps to reject them? Does that mean you are throwing these "gifts" back in God's face? Please understand the nature of a "gift." It is not something that is crammed forcibly down the throat of the recipient.

According to the conservative version of Christian tradition embraced by "born again" evangelicals, the greatest "gift" from God was salvation offered by the grace of Jesus. Should Christian believers feel entitled to enact **legislation** to require by **force of**

90

law that everyone be required to proclaim their acceptance of Jesus as savior?

Isaiah 49:15: "Can a woman forget her sucking child, that she should not have compassion on the son of her womb? yea, they may forget, yet will I not forget thee." (KJV)

This scripture isn't even talking about fetal life. It is referring to the relationship of God to the Children of Israel, using the metaphor of born children, already sucking. The reference to "womb" is where he came from, not where he is or who he is now. Use of this scripture in relevance to abortion is very far from its actual context and, in any case, it would have been a perfect opportunity to condemn abortion, but no such condemnation or prohibition is here.

This verse would actually be better applied to those who claim to be "Christian," yet defend the lives of unborn *potential* children while turning away hungry or sick children of disadvantage.

Luke 1:36,41: "[36] And, behold, thy cousin Elisabeth, she hath also conceived a son in her old age: and this is the sixth month with her, who was called barren. [41] And it came to pass, that, when Elisabeth heard the salutation of Mary, the babe leaped in her womb; and Elisabeth was filled with the Holy Ghost." (KJV)

This scripture contains the words of the angel to Mary, informing her of Elisabeth's pregnancy, already in the sixth month (3rd trimester); Mary's visit occurs sometime after that — so we know that this is well past quickening and normal fetal movement, and even well past the point where purely elective abortion is allowed or practiced anywhere in the United States.

In this situation, with God's and others' foreknowledge, there is an awareness that the two fetuses discussed will, in fact, go beyond "potential" to become actual human beings of unique and special greatness.

In any case, the examples of John the Baptist and Jesus Christ, as two of the most exceptional figures in the Christian message, are hardly the basis for establishing general rules that apply to the routine lives of ordinary people and their daily situations. Special cases rarely serve as good models for general rules.

That said, however, there is certainly nothing here about first trimester pregnancies (when most abortions occur) since both Mary and Elisabeth are already well beyond that point in this passage, or anything that even remotely suggests that a first trimester embryo has a soul, or equal status as a human.

And even if it did, there is still not a single denunciation of abortion in the Bible — again, this would have been a perfect opportunity for comment on the subject of abortion if there was any such intent, and *the Bible writers intentionally remain silent.*

Exodus 20:13: "Thou shalt not kill." (KJV)

This scripture in Exodus 20:13 from the Ten Commandments is often translated in more modern versions as "Thou shalt not commit murder."

One could easily look at the Ten Commandments and view them as something of an "index" to the Law of Moses which follows in the remainder of Exodus, Leviticus and Deuteronomy.

Each of the Ten Commandments, from the rituals by which we show love of God and eschew idols or "other gods," defining taking the Name of the Lord in vain, or how we honor our parents, etc., is defined in more detail elsewhere in the Law.

Considering that the Bible, including other sections of the Law of Moses, also present numerous situations in where killing is not only permitted but commanded, to imply that this summary point prohibits all taking of life is to claim that every other part of the Bible that allows or even requires it creates an internal contradiction.

In the same way, "murder" is carefully defined elsewhere in Exodus, Leviticus and Deuteronomy as to details regarding relationships and situations (but not methods) and including the specific penalty for each class of murder. And none of those who claim a Biblical basis for claiming that abortion is murder are ever able to cite which of the penalties applies to abortion.

Those details specifically omit any reference to abortion, while covering other subjects at an equivalent level of specificity, so it is very dishonest to try and apply it to abortion any more than to self-defense — a woman defending her body against an unwanted "invader" in cases where that new life is not desired.

It is interesting to note that the Bible defines in detail many types of both justifiable (self-defense, executions, wartime) and criminal killing (various types of homicides and relationships to those killed — strangers, neighbors, Israelites, family members, etc.) are discussed, along with any applicable penalties.

Even when the subject of the fetus' existence or death comes up, it still does not prohibit the well-known practice of abortion. So, obviously it was not an oversight, either in the original pronouncements or the failure of the later prophets, Jesus or the apostles to clarify.

The Bible neither promotes nor discourages abortion. Period. The intentional omission of prohibitions against abortion obviously mean they intended that to be left to personal choice, unless one believes God made a mistake.

Such a simplistic and simple-minded definition of this blanket statement, the commandment "thou shalt not kill," with no other qualification, could also be cited to prohibit vaccinations that **kill** *millions* of viruses or bacteria to save one human (the statement does not specifically mention that it applies only to killing humans); it could prohibit killing shrimp, lobster, fish, birds and mammals to satisfy the lust for artery-clogging animal fat. If one claims that it only means *human* life, then this blanket statement would prohibit still killing sperms, eggs, or even adult humans in situations of self-defense, in wartime or for executions. However, no one who understands the ten commandments, not even vegetarians, would claim such blanket authority from Exodus 20:13.

Unlike these other subsets to non-excepted principles, killing is defined at a level to which classes are identified — and *some* are prohibited while others are *permitted* (killing of animals, killing humans in self defense) and some are mandated (killing of humans in wartime, lawful execution for crimes including many acts such as adultery, accusations of "witchcraft," worshipping other deities, working on the Sabbath or even talking back to parents).

In other words, at the level of detail definition that would have included abortion, there are both prohibitions *and* exceptions to the rule, so at this level of specificity the principle is *not* applicable to non-excepted subsets, unless you include abortion as a subset woman's self defense of her body, in which case it becomes specifically *permitted* by the umbrella principle.

The Bible offers various statements about fetal movement after quickening, as well as references to the physical formation of fetal development. It is interesting to note that, if the Bible's silence on abortion in the Law of Moses had been an oversight (does God make oversights?) these many subsequent references by the prophets, or later clarification of the Law by Jesus or the apostles in their epistles, gave many excellent opportunities to clarify their intent against the well-known practice of abortion, if they had intended scripture to condemn it. Discussions of fetal formation, life and movement would have been a perfect opportunity to condemn abortion — *if* the Bible or any of the Bible writers ever had any such intent. *But they didn't.*

Exodus 21:22: "If men strive, and hurt a woman with child, so that her fruit depart [from her], and yet no mischief follow: he shall be surely punished, according as the woman's husband will lay upon him; and he shall pay as the judges [determine]." (KJV)

Note to those who try to construe this passage into somehow opposing the right of a woman (or her husband, in the days before women had many rights) to voluntarily choose to have an abortion.

This scripture has nothing to do with the voluntary, intentional choice of a woman (or her husband). It is about two men struggling together who *accidentally* cause a woman to have a miscarriage, and the resulting penalties. The point is that this verse is about third-party causation rather than voluntary choice.

Without trying to equate human tissue with property, it is more analogous to someone voluntarily disposing of unwanted property (no problem) as opposed to a third party taking it against the owner's will (theft).

Even so, notice that the value here is on the *woman,* not the fetus. The penalties vary, depending on whether or not there is "harm."

Harm? To whom?

The fetus?

In the passage, there has already been a miscarriage — by definition *the fetus is already dead*. The variability of "harm" obviously means injury to the woman. But even if there is no harm (injury) they must still have a penalty because, like modern fundamentalists wish to do, they deprived her (or her husband) of *choice* (in this case, to complete a pregnancy).

This example of a third-party violent attack (or carelessness) on another person has no relevance whatsoever to the situation in which a woman makes a *voluntary* choice to abort the contents of her *own body* under *medically-supervised conditions*.

The fact that this example is even raised regarding something it has no relation to shows the abject desperation of those who want to find something, anything, in the Bible, but who cannot find anything that actually says what they want it to. They need to just accept the Bible as it is, or just write their own the way they want it to be.

Psalm 139:13-16: "[13] For thou hast possessed my reins: thou hast covered me in my mother's womb. [14] I will praise thee; for I am fearfully [and] wonderfully made: marvelous [are] thy works; and [that] my soul knoweth right well. [15] My substance was not hid from thee, when I was made in secret, [and] curiously wrought in the lowest parts of the earth. [16] Thine eyes did see my substance, yet being unperfect; and in thy book all [my members] were written, [which] in continuance were fashioned, when [as yet there was] none of them." (KJV)

This scripture describes the purely physical process of bodily formation, a process that everyone knows is occurring in utero. Here is a perfect opportunity for a later prophet to also confirm that a soul is also attached to these purely physical body parts (cell tissues) of "unformed substance," and clarify any ambiguity in the supposedly "perfect" Law of Moses, yet no such clarification is forthcoming.

The context here is that Psalms 139 is David's praise to the Lord, written as the lyrics to music. Here David is praising God, not commenting on embryology and, in any case, says nothing about the soul or humanity of the embryo.

Genesis 9:6-7: "[6] Whoso sheddeth man's blood, by man shall his blood be shed: for in the image of God made he man. [7] And you, be ye fruitful, and multiply; bring forth abundantly in the earth, and multiply therein." (KJV) [Compare Genesis 1:28]

In this scripture, verse six clearly refers to human life. If the fetus or embryo is not yet a human person, this clearly does not apply. If one wants to be literal, it refers to killing a man. Not even women or children! Certainly it is not referring to mere human genetic tissue — hair, fingernails, other organs, pre-human potentially-developing tissue. The passage does not mention abortion here or anywhere else. Later, in giving the law (Exodus, Leviticus, Deuteronomy) forms of killing that are acceptable and

98

unacceptable are spelled out in detail, with varying punishments and consequences for various forms of forbidden killing. Abortion is never mentioned once. It is neither promoted nor prohibited. The Bible is completely neutral; it is left to individual human choice.

Verse seven is a command to "Be fertile, then, and multiply." The commandment to "multiply and replenish the earth and subdue it" is a very specific command to a specific group of people, given only twice in the Bible: once to Adam and Eve at the start of the human race (Gen 1:28), and again to Noah and his family when they are the only human survivors after the Great Flood (Gen 9:7) and are tasked with repopulating the Earth.

In both of these specific situations, there is a severe population shortage. Clearly the context is to build up the human species. The command has been obeyed. The earth is filled with people. Many today would argue that we have been not only fruitful, but way beyond that. The earth has been subdued.

Adam and Eve, and later Noah and his family of flood survivors, were told to have "dominion" over the earth. To have "dominion" does not mean to destroy. The same word, "dominion," is used throughout the Bible to describe a husband's relationship to his wife and children, but while the Bible is certainly chauvinistic and patriarchal in favoring male authority, it does not equate this dominion with destroying them; rather to conserve and protect that which is precious.

This command was given specifically to Adam and Eve and to Noah and his family when they were the only people on earth. It was very specific and narrowly focused, like other individual commandments telling a specific person to go to this place or perform a specific action.

The command to multiply was never repeated again to any other people (as other commandments that are repeated over and over), nor was it ever included in any generalized codification of commandments, nor was it needed by any other people. And since abortion has been known and practiced by all peoples in all times (whether legal or not), we can look at the great population of the human family and see that abortion has hardly stood in the way of our species being "fruitful."

Genesis 2:7: "Then the LORD God formed man of dust from the ground, and breathed into his nostrils the breath of life; and man became a living being." (KJV)

This passage describe the creation and ensoulment of Adam, the first human. Here ensoulment clearly is defined in the Bible as occurring *after* the taking of "first breath." And please note that the reference equating "ensoulment" and "breath of life" can be found not only in this reference to the special creation of Adam, but throughout both Old and New Testaments, applying to all the rest of us. Clearly the concept of ensoulment beginning with the first breath taken is a general doctrine, not merely specific to the unique case of Adam.

Numbers 5:12-28: And last, but certainly not least, we absolutely need to cite the one passage in the Bible that the anti-choice extremists will never tell you about.

While the Bible never forbids (nor encourages) abortion, there is one passage from the Law of Moses that can be interpreted as authorizing abortion in the case of a married woman who is suspected of committing adultery and therefore might become impregnated by a man other than her husband.

This passage says that if a man suspects his wife to have been unfaithful (and thus subject to becoming pregnant by someone else), he can take her to the priest who will prescribe the "bitter water," that the Hebrews believed to be an abortifacient produced by combining pennyroyal with black cohosh, for a potion that will magically indicate whether she is innocent or guilty of the offense. Oh, and by the way, this potion was also believed to be something that could terminate any unwanted pregnancy that might also have existed.

Note that this is part of the Law of Moses. This is not a specific instance to a particular individual or couple. This was a general prescription of practice for God's "Chosen People" — the Jews — from whom the promised Messiah was supposed to appear.

The reference is this passage is to the Hebrew ritual of Sotah, using an ancient abortifacient of "bitter water" described in the King James Version as "ephah of barley meal."

The ritual is required in cases where a man suspects that his wife may have been impregnated by another man. According to the Hebrews' superstitions about the ritual of Sotah, if the woman were guilty, any possible bastard fetus would be expelled (aborted), but would remain safe if she were innocent.

While abortion per se is not mentioned here or anywhere else in the Bible, the references to Sotah causing "thy high to rot, and thy belly to swell," as well as the "curse" to a woman (the loss of a pregnancy or the barrenness of total infertility), may not be clearly understood by many readers in our time, but would be clearly understood in the era in which it was written. There are many non-scriptural accounts showing how herbal abortifacients were employed, using herbal methods such as combining pennyroyal with black cohosh or blue cohosh [more detailed accounts and precise methods can be found by going to any search engine, such as Google and typing in as required key words: "cohosh blue black pennyroyal abortion"].

Historical religious views

Early Hebrew Views

The Talmud, a core foundational interpretive text of Rabbinical Judaism whose earliest passages date back to Old Testament times, has generally been seen as being pro-choice.

The following are exact quotes from p. 238 of the Steinsaltz Edition of the Talmud, translated by Rabbi Israel V. Berman, 1989 edition (published by Random House):

"A fetus is [considered as] the thigh of its mother, i.e., it is like a limb of the mother, and is not a separate entity."

"A human fetus [is] less than a fully undependent human being."

"A fetus cannot inherit property until it is born."

The twelfth century Jewish rabbi Maimonides, one of the premier influences in the development of modern Jewish understanding, taught that these Talmudic passages in conjunction with the Biblical passages in Exodus 21:22, along with the "first breath" concept (as in Adam) [Genesis 2:7] permitted abortion until the baby's head had emerged. (His work, "The Guide of the Perplexed," completed in 1190, blended Jewish thought with the teachings of Aristotle. The work was so highly regarded that it was also embraced by other non-Jewish theologians, and was even cited by St. Thomas Aquinas as a seminal source.)

Christian-era Non-Biblical opposition to abortion

In fairness, while there were early works that accepted the right of women (or at least their husbands) to abort unwanted pregnancies, there are also early Christian writings that spoke out in opposition to elective abortion.

Here are some of the early *non-biblical* references often cited by conservative Christians opposing abortion dating back to the early Christian era:

Sibylline Oracles 2, pg. 339

Didache, Chapter 2 verse 3

Letter to Barnabus from the Codex Sinaiticus from unknown author

Letter to Diognetus [Epistle of Mathetes to Diognetus dates to around 130 A.D. — citation Chapter 5:6]

While it is absolutely necessary to acknowledge that some early Christians did oppose abortion, several key points also become equally clear and have to be acknowledged:

1. Those in Biblical times *did know* about abortion, so the Bible's silence on abortion cannot be excused on the basis that they didn't know about it. However, since God supposedly breathed the inspiration for the Bible and he supposedly *did know* everything, even that should have been no excuse. Since God could see the future, including the future controversy about this issue, the decision not to provide a simple, clear, unambiguous statement proactively preventing that controversy must have been intentional.

2. The passages that opposed abortion were **not included** in the Bible. While several of these texts were considered for inclusion in the Canon, not one of these opportunities to include a clear statement of Biblical opposition to abortion was accepted. Any effort to have the Bible unambiguously oppose abortion *was rejected!*

3. Nothing that actually made it into the Bible opposes abortion.

The simple fact is that the Bible is completely silent about abortion. The Bible does not encourage or promote abortion nor does it discourage or oppose abortion in any way. It is completely neutral, therefore leaving that up to each individual person to make their own personal *choice*.

But believe it or not, I have had people respond by asking, "Well, then, where in the Bible does it say that abortion is *permitted?*"

Such a comment somehow suggests that everything is *forbidden* unless God specifically OK's it. Where in the Bible does it say that it is permitted to use a computer, drive a motorized vehicle, fly in the air, inoculate against disease (and thus kill billions of God's creations — the viruses and bacteria)? [I am not comparing zygotes to viruses, merely showing how silly it is to make such a ridiculous assertion.]

Oh, these things weren't invented yet?

You don't think that God (who knew Jeremiah before the foundation of the world) could foresee the future day?

Whatever the reason, those things are still not specifically authorized. What about things that were known? Where in the Bible does it say it's OK to climb a tree? Kill a shrimp or pig for dinner (I can show you where it is *forbidden)?*

The only rational presumption is to conclude that what is not prohibited (either directly or by inclusion in a subset of what is prohibited) is permitted.

Abortion was known and practiced in Bible times. And there are lots of other things that were within the scope of technology for Bible times, but not authorized by the Bible: is surfing allowed by the Bible?

Are competitive team sports authorized in scripture?

Picnics? Climbing trees? Going to the zoo?

The Bible is completely silent about abortion. Neutral. The Bible neither supports, encourages, condemns nor discourages the practice. It is left to individual discretion ... or *choice*. As to whether abortion should be *legal*, as discussed at length in Chapter Two, my view takes the balance of the middle ground: the far left (Chinese Communists) want forced abortion mandated by law; the far right (Christian Conservatives) want forced pregnancy mandated by law; the middle ground (Moderate Middle) leaves it up to each individual ... *just like the Bible.*

Ensoulment

Can more than one soul inhabit the same body? If one believes that only one soul can inhabit a body, then what happens in the case of identical multiple births?

Each twin or triplet has its own soul at birth and is its own person.

Yet at the time of fertilization / conception, there was only one cell, one entity and one unique genetic individual. One must conclude either that multiple souls can inhabit a body, or that the soul has not yet come to exist at the time (after conception / fertilization) of the division into multiples.

Let's compare the development of a *home* to the development of an *ensouled human person.*

The owner is like the ovum. The architect is like the sperm. The owner (egg) has the complete resources to build a home, including the ideas of how it should take place, but lacks the precise finishing of the plans for doing so.

The architect (sperm) replaces those vague, general ideas with a more technically viable representation, infusing his own new additional thoughts and ideas. The resources/ideas of the owner come together with the technical specifications of the architect, and the result of this union is a complete blueprint, or set of building plans (a fertilized zygote).

These plans now have to be implanted to an actual construction site, provided by the owner. Even after actual construction has begun, there is nothing yet resembling a HOME.

The framing rapidly takes shape and soon begins to resemble the form of a home, though there are no actual walls, insulation, pipes or wiring yet. Even as construction progresses and the wiring and plumbing are added, there still is not a home. Even in the final stages of construction, it *looks like* a home, but no one lives there. It does not actual become a home until a family moves into it (ensoulment) and gives it the spiritual warmth that distinguishes a **home** from a **house**.

While there are many references in the Bible to ensoulment of those who have been born, and many references to conception, birth and pregnancy, there is not one single Bible verse that indicates that ensoulment occurs prior to the taking of first breath.

Believe it or not, some have responded by asking me to show evidence that ensoulment did not occur at conception or during pregnancy. One of the most basic principles in Logic 101 is that it is impossible to prove a negative (i.e., that there is not a soul). The person asserting an affirmative claim (i.e., that there *is* a soul) is the one with the burden of proving that assertion. I am not making the positive assertion of when ensoulment occurs, or even if such a thing exists. Those who claim that it occurs at or before a certain point are the ones required to prove the claim they assert.

Recommended reading:

Additional recommended resources regarding the history of abortion during Bible times:

J. Ricci, *The Genealogy of Gynaecology* 52, 84, 113, 149 (2d ed. 1950).

L. Lader, *Abortion* 75-77 (1966)

K. Niswander, *Medical Abortion Practices in the United States*, in Abortion and the Law 37, 38-40 (D. Smith ed. 1967)

G. Williams, *The Sanctity of Life and the Criminal Law* 148 (1957)

J. Noonan, *An Almost Absolute Value in History, in The Morality of Abortion* 1, 3-7 (J. Noonan ed. 1970)

Quay, *Justifiable Abortion - Medical and Legal Foundations* (pt. 2), 49 Geo. L. J. 395, 406-422 (1961) (hereinafter Quay).

Tribe, Laurence (Constitutional Law professor at Harvard) *Abortion: The Clash of Absolutes* (section on history) 1990:Norton.

Special note: I would like to express appreciation to Davis D. Danizier ("3D") for assistance in compiling the religious perspective and, in particular, the scriptural documentation.

Dave is the author of the excellent book *Betrayal of Jesus* which, along with his web pages, present his own important contribution to the demystification of Christian mythology. The website can be found at: http://danizier.wordpress.com/

4

ＡDDITIONAL ＩSSUES:
ＬATE-ＴERM, ＰARENTAL ＣONSENT, ＲAPE

This chapter addresses other popular issues and additional aspects that are often brought up regarding the issues related to abortion that don't fit neatly into the more specific issues of the previous chapters, based on the morality of when human *life* becomes human *person,* the legal issues or the religious aspects of the issue.

Some of these additional issues include discussions of late-term abortion (extremely rare and only done under conditions of extreme medical trauma), demands for parental consent before a minor can obtain an abortion, abortion in cases of rape and incest, comparisons of abortion to the Holocaust or slavery, the dishonesty of graphic posters and signs,

111

the myth of abortion-induced guilt, and other issues in women's reproductive self-determination.

Late Term Abortion

The reality of late-term abortion is that it is extremely rare — fewer than four out of 10,000 abortions, according to figures from the Centers for Disease Control.

Late term abortion is used almost exclusively to terminate pregnancies that were wanted, but in which something has gone very wrong, late in the process. Many of those who have late term abortions are traumatized twice: once in the loss of a *wanted* pregnancy, and again in being demonized by cruel individuals trying to promote a religious agenda no matter how many lives they destroy or how many people they hurt.

Some of the worst cruelty and bullying has occurred by those protesting and obstructing against women obtaining late-term abortions of pregnancies they wanted, already traumatized by but which went terribly wrong.

I have seen televised interviews or videos of televised testimony before legislative bodies in which women who had been carrying much-wanted pregnancies, and some who had even been previously opposed to abortion, who were forced by tragic circumstances to have to surgically terminate wanted but failed pregnancies. They testified through tears, both for much-wanted potentials that were lost and then for the cruelty they had to endure when they were villainized.

These very rare personal, private tragedies are being exploited by those opposed to women's reproductive self-determination as a means of demonizing all abortions, including first-term abortions (when almost 90% of all abortions actually occur) which have little if any resemblance to abortions in late term.

Abortion and Rape

No person who denies the right of women to terminate an unwanted pregnancy that results from rape can ever raise the issue that a woman should make her "choice" prior to consenting to pregnancy since rape, by definition, precludes consent.

And no, pregnancy resulting from rape is not "rare." It happens tens of thousands of times ever year. And no, it is not a "gift from god," sorry, Richard Mourdock, failed Indiana candidate for the U.S. Senate. And the tens of thousands of rape pregnancies every year prove that, no, the female body does not have a way to "shut that whole thing down and, no, there is no such thing as a "legitimate rape" (sorry, Todd Aiken, failed Missouri candidate for the U.S. Senate).

The fact is, any rape can and does result in pregnancy.

Abortion, Rape and Contemporary Politics

In the 2016 campaign for president of the United States, Republican primary candidates doubled down on their efforts to stake out the most extreme positions in forcing rape victims to bear the offspring of their attackers. In an unprecedented field of seventeen announced candidates, virtually all Republican candidates took positions opposing a woman's right to choose to terminate an unwanted pregnancy.

The more moderate candidates would permit abortions in cases of rape, incest or to save the life of the mother. The most extreme candidates, including Ted Cruz, Marco Rubio, Mike Huckabee and Scott Walker, all took hard-line positions against allowing women to make the most personal decisions about the most private parts of their bodies, even when those bodies are at risk of death or were invaded by the assaults of rapists.

And then they all scratched their heads and wondered why people thought their party was waging a "war against women."

Abortion, Rape and Consent to Pregnancy

Some anti-choice extremists try to argue that women should not be able to choose to abort an unwanted pregnancy resulting from consensual sex, because they consented to pregnancy when they consented to sex, knowing that pregnancy was a possible outcome of that choice.

That argument is, of course, absurd to begin with, as discussed at length in Chapter One: "Moral Issues: Life vs. Personhood." Consent to sexual intimacy is no more consent to an unwanted pregnancy, even though it is a known possible outcome, than consent to riding in a car is consent to the known possible outcome of an automobile accident.

But even those who labor under that deluded mis-understanding of consent as a basis for general opposition to abortion, cannot raise that issue in cases where pregnancy results from rape. One cannot cite the consent issue as a generalized basis for opposing abortion, and then dispute the right to abort in situations in which no such consent to that sexual assault exists in the first place.

And the question of rape is not just something women can relate to. When discussing rape, men need to remember that even men can also be raped, and not just in prisons. And while this is rare, and the numbers of victims are overwhelmingly female, I would never wish such a personal violation on anyone, including those who demonstrate a lack of empathy for the victims of rape.

To anyone who bears no compassion for the victims of rape, I really want you to actually, seriously think about this and how *you* would feel if the most private part of *your* body were penetrated by an unwanted assailant against your will.

Parental Notification and Parental Consent

Many of those who oppose abortion seek to restrict access by enacting laws that require any underage girl carrying an unwanted pregnancy should be prohibited from obtaining an abortion until her parent(s) or other guardian(s) are notified and have given their consent for that procedure.

Most who support women's rights to reproductive self-determination believe that a girl who is old enough to be pregnant is old enough to make certain decisions that affect the rest of *her* life and which *she* more than anyone else will bear consequences for the rest of her life.

I have never seen a "parental notification and consent" proposal that includes a requirement that the parents who make a decision opposing their daughter's choice to abort are then required to assume lifetime liability for responsibility and support of the child resulting from their overriding decision.

The flip side overlooked by those opposed to choice: And how would the anti-choice conservatives feel about the flip side of that situation. An underage girl gets pregnant, ignores the lifetime consequences of a choice to become a mother, and decides she wants to carry the pregnancy to term and keep the resulting baby. The parents think she is too young to become a mother. The parents think this will close doors to education, opportunity and a chance to just be a normal teenager, and that such a choice ruin her life. The parents believe an abortion would be the best way to handle a problem situation, but a girl wants to carry to term. Do those who support mandatory parental consent also agree that the will of the parents should prevail when their choice is to abort rather than complete a pregnancy?

Some point out that a girl can get an abortion to terminate an unwanted pregnancy without telling her parents, but can't get an aspirin without parental permission. We are not talking about headaches and aspirin here, but life-changing consequences, regarding an issue that is loaded with emotional and moral implications and long-term results that don't apply to taking an aspirin to relieve a headache that will go away by itself.

An underage girl may not be old enough to make all adult decisions, or to consent to legal adult choices or even adult relationships, but if she is pregnant, the choice — with all its life-changing consequences — as to whether she aborts, carries or gives the child up for adoption, should be hers.

It is the girl who will be the one who endures the consequences for the rest of her life. That is true whether she was forcibly raped, the victim of incest or "thought" she was in love and was trying to act like the adult that she isn't. In any case, the examples of incest and child abuse are, alone, valid reasons why notification laws are not workable.

The issue of parental notification and consent goes beyond mere parental authority or the parent-child relationship. Almost all girls with a problem situation will turn first to their parents for help. They may be nervous, or fearful, or uncomfortable, but when they get in that situation, it is almost always their parents who will be the first adult authorities they turn to. In the case where a girl can't go to her parents with this kind of problem, then she should not have to. The very fact that she feels this inability to go to her parents in a way that most girls readily would, already raises red flags about the family dynamics.

And the alternative is what? A scared teenage girl being forced to go to a judge? A scared teenage girl who can't go to her parents going to an imposing, authoritative stranger who may be pushing his or her own ideological values?

The whole point of requiring parental consent and notification is to set up one more roadblock to make abortion harder. Newsflash! Unless the teenage girl intends to perform her own "do it yourself" abortion, she *is* going to be talking to adult professionals, even in the extremely rare instances when she can't go to her parents. The whole point of having *legal* abortion rights is so women don't need to have a "do it yourself" or back-alley job. Look at the reality. This issue is not about parental control; if she can't go to her parents with this kind of problem at this age, the parents have already lost control. It is all about stopping girls from having abortions at all.

The Myth of Abortion-induced Guilt

One of the enduring myths about abortion is that women who have one will be emotionally scarred. The reality is quite different.

Millions of women have had abortions, many more than one. The vast majority of these women have no regrets, and almost all report that it was the right choice for them at that time and in that situation. The reality is that a routine first trimester abortion, such as 90% of abortions, is quick, painless and medically safe. In fact, there is less medical risk from abortion than from nine months of full term pregnancy followed by childbirth.

Very few women express regrets, and numerous studies spanning decades as cited below have consistently confirmed that roughly nine out of ten feel no subsequent guilt or regret at all.

The few instances where regret occurs can be traced to situations in either of two situations: First, other people (parent, husband, boyfriend, religious advisor, religious peer community, etc.) pressure a woman to make a choice that was *not* her own freely-made choice. Or second, women later converted to religious beliefs that imposed external guilt on them that they did not experience before such conversion and would not otherwise have experienced without that self-fulfilling prophecy.

Unless imposed externally by pressures to make an unwanted choice, or by artificially-manufactured religious guilt, self-generated remorse from abortion is almost entirely nonexistent.

L.A. Times: 1-27-2011 p. A8: "Abortion does not prompt mental problems, study finds" by Shari Roan http://articles.latimes.com/2011/jan/26/health/la-he-abortion-20110127

San Diego Union-Tribune 1-27-2011 p. A15: "No higher mental health risk after abortion, study finds" by Alicia Chang, Associated Press http://www.signonsandiego.com/news/2011/jan/26/stu dy-no-higher-mental-health-risk-after-abortion/

Base source: New England Journal of Medicine 1-27-2011

http://www.nejm.org/doi/full/10.1056/NEJMoa0905882

Consistent with 2008 study by Linda Beckman conducted by: American Psychological Association: "Mental Health and Abortion" by Brenda Major, PhD, Chair, Mark Appelbaum, PhD, Linda Beckman, PhD, Mary Ann Dutton, PhD, Nancy Felipe Russo, PhD, Carolyn West, PhD, August 2008 http://www.apa.org/pi/women/programs/abortion/index.aspx

Comparing Abortion to the Holocaust

Some people try to equate the widespread exercise by women of control over their own bodies with the systematic genocidal attempt to exterminate Jewish populations in Nazi Germany by Adolf Hitler. Not only is this an absurd attempt at false equivalence, but it is highly insulting to Jewish people.

There are several big differences:

Jewish people had measurable EEG brain waves and actual thoughts, feelings, emotions and sentience. Fetuses do not.

Jewish people were *not* occupying the most private part of someone else's body.

Comparing the value of a living, breathing, sentient Jew to that of a speck of embryonic tissue is a tremendously anti-Semitic insult to a people who have been persecuted enough.

In the Holocaust they killed real, live, conscious and feeling human beings, with individual experience and personal histories. A first trimester abortion removes cell tissue that has no sensation or awareness or thoughts or feelings or experience of any kind. Zero. Not even any measurable EEG brain waves. The differences between human *life* (which begins *before* fertilization — the sperm and egg were alive and of the human species, ergo, "human life," long before that milestone) and human person) and being a human *person,* are discussed at length in Chapter One: "Moral Issues: Life vs. Personhood."

But even if a fetus *were* a human person, it would not have the right to dominate the body of someone else and demand 24-hour care for 9 months from a woman against her will; after birth the baby is pretty helpless, but constant, ongoing care from a specific caregiver is not required.

Anyone who can reduce sentient, autonomous Jewish human persons to nothing more than the equivalent of insentient fetal tissue with no brain waves is anti-Semitic.

Comparing Abortion to Slavery

Anti-choice conservatives also frequently try to equate allowing women the freedom to control their own bodies with the inhumanity of denying liberty to other human beings impressed into slavery.

In their absurd reversal of reality, they try to equate denying freedom for African American slaves with allowing freedom for women.

As with the absurdity of those who try to invoke the Holocaust, such false equivalence demeans the real victims. Saying there is no moral difference between the horrible human rights abuses of fully human slaves of African ancestry and undeveloped, pre-sentient human cell tissue is a terrible cultural offense against the victims of slavery and their descendants. Maybe white males just don't feel enough compassion for the victims of slavery, mostly from other racial backgrounds, or the victims of anti-choice policies, who are mostly women.

For all the reasons discussed in Chapter One: "Moral Issues: Life vs. Personhood," the fetus is not a full *actual* human person, but pre-sentient human tissue that has the *potential* to grow into a human person if certain conditions are met.

And *even if the pre-natal uterine contents were a human person,* it would not have the right to demand control of another person's body against her will. Imagine a hypothetical court case involving two estranged brothers. One had two healthy kidneys, the other's kidneys had failed and he needed a transplant in order to survive. They were genetically compatible, but the healthy brother refused to give up one of his kidneys. The sick brother — a fully-human person — sued in court to force the organ donation, saying he had an inalienable right to life. The court rightly agreed that, while voluntary organ donation is a beautiful choice, people cannot be *forced* to keep someone else alive by using their bodies *against their will.*

The closest similarity to slavery applicable to the issue of abortion is the attempt to deny a woman's right to prevent a fetus from *controlling her body against her will* and *making her a ... slave.*

As I have said, the only relevant comparison between the issues of slavery and abortion is that of sentient being (Black slave) to sentient being (woman) who are both forced to have their bodies used for the interests of others against their will.

Please remember, the modern women's rights movement began at the 1848 (pre-Civil War) World Anti-Slavery Convention in London, when Elizabeth Cady Stanton and Lucretia Mott — women — were refused participation because of their gender. The two women quickly realized that, in that time, women were being oppressed in much the same way as slaves. They decided their first priority should be to free the women before trying to get active in trying to free the slaves.

Graphic Posters and Signs

Who are the deceptive ones carrying gross signs with graphic pictures of aborted fetuses around schools and clinics to *force* people to see such pictures?

The pictures themselves are deceptive and dishonest. They usually show pictures of late-term fetuses (less than four out of 10,000 abortions occur in the third trimester, and only for extreme conditions of extreme trauma) in a general campaign against all abortions (89% of which occur in the first trimester). They have to do this, of course, because if they showed pictures of an embryo at the stage when routine abortions are actually performed, the barely visible, primitive life form would not register the kind of revulsion they seek to evoke.

Since they can't convince people on the merits of serious argument, the anti-choice extremists who use such tactics have just one hope: to try to gross people out with pictures dripping with as much blood and gore as they can fit on a poster, and then parade them where small children will be present. In *my* community, such tactics have backfired, and even many of the less extreme opponents of abortion have expressed their outrage and revulsion.

Many medical procedures are gruesome. Should we show posters of open-heart surgeries to small children? Or pictures of people whose faces are being reconstructed after grotesque auto accidents?

The more extreme elements of the pro-life movement don't care about women as human persons. They only care about fetal tissue. Should vegetarians parade in front of restaurants where patrons are dining meals that include meat, with pictures of what goes on in the slaughterhouse where their meal came from?

Planned Parenthood

Planned Parenthood was founded by a feminist who opposed abortion and believed that widespread access to birth control would be the best way to reduce the number of abortions. Today, Planned Parenthood has evolved to support full reproductive freedom for women, yet even now less than 3% of Planned Parenthood's operations involve abortion.

On its face, therefore, the subject of Planned Parenthood should have little to do with the issue of abortion. But since there is so much widespread opposition to Planned Parenthood based on the inaccurate perception of Planned Parenthood as an abortion provider, many opponents of women's reproductive choice repeatedly bring up the subject of Planned Parenthood when discussing abortion-related issues. And when they do, these conservatives almost always distort and misrepresent the facts about Planned Parenthood — what their operations are and how those operations are carried out.

Common Misrepresentations

Planned Parenthood operations: Planned Parenthood is often depicted as some kind of abortion mill. This is simply inaccurate and does injustice to the full range of medical services offered.

Contrary to popular mythology based on intentional misrepresentations by those who oppose women's access to medical care, Planned Parenthood is not primarily a provider of abortions. While there are certainly some wonderful medical providers who do specialize in access to abortion services for women, and there is nothing wrong with that, to describe Planned Parenthood as an abortion mill is simply not accurate.

In fact, at the time it was founded, the founder was opposed to abortion and believed that access to birth control would reduce the number of abortions. No abortions were offered, and even today, while Planned Parenthood has evolved its views and now supports women's rights of reproductive choice, many local centers do not directly provide abortion services at all, though they will refer to other facilities that do offer a more complete range of options in dealing with unwanted pregnancies.

For women, Planned Parenthood offers birth control (which is the single most effective tool for preventing unwanted pregnancies and thus the need to consider abortion), family counseling, fertility services, prevention and treatment of sexually-transmitted diseases, mammograms, cancer screenings and many other medical services. As for abortion, the reality is that abortions are only performed through a limited number of facilities and account for less than 3% of Planned Parenthood's operations.

And for men, while Planned Parenthood originally concentrated on reproductive services for women, today Planned Parenthood also provides medical and reproductive services for men in their Men's Clinic. Such services include vasectomies as well as prevention and treatment for sexually-transmitted diseases and the treatment and prevention of erectile dysfunction. Some of the non-gender-specific medical screenings that are available for women may also be available for men.

Other misrepresentations: In many cases, those seeking to discredit Planned Parenthood and undermine its funding from both public and private sources have been so desperate that they have simply *fib*ricated false evidence to support claims that they felt would be sufficiently outrage in the court of public opinion, even though they were based entirely on misrepresentations.

One of the most egregious was the 2015 release of a serious of "undercover" videos intended to show what they claimed was Planned Parenthood representatives engaged in negotiating the most favorable prices for the sale of organs and other body tissues from late-term abortions for research or organ donations.

The videos were heavily edited to misrepresent the totality of the exchanges, including addition of material not even from Planned Parenthood, or distorted to misrepresent the context of what was being said, and were presented as drawing conclusions contrary to actual facts.

Aside from the fact that abortions after the first trimester are extremely rare, the fact is that Planned Parenthood does not sell fetal organs or tissues at all. Such activities would be illegal and, if the videos had the slightest bit of credibility, you can be certain that anti-choice conservatives would be aggressive in prosecuting such crimes.

No such prosecutions have occurred.

However if a woman requests that fetal organs or tissues be donated rather than discarded, she has the right to request, with a written and signed consent form, that such tissue she provides be so donated. And when that occurs, Planned Parenthood can request appropriate reimbursement of its actual costs from the facilities that receive such donated tissue. There is no profit, only the direct reimbursement of actual costs.

In some cases the facilities receiving the tissue are for-profit businesses and do make money off their services, but Planned Parenthood does not.

Those who recorded the videos misrepresented their identities and affiliations, misrepresented the full context of dialogue and presented highly-edited final videos that were extremely dishonest and even included material completely unrelated to Planned Parenthood.

The bottom line is that Planned Parenthood is a comprehensive non-profit provider of medical services. To the minimal extent that it provides abortions, it is a very small part of what they do.

Margaret Sanger and the founding of Planned Parenthood

Critics of Planned Parenthood often bring up the name of Margaret Founder, a courageous champion of women's rights and advocate of birth control who founded Planned Parenthood.

These critics cite, often with great misrepresentation (when attempting to respond to such people, it is advisable to always verify quotes and sources independently as there is a great deal of misrepresentation being thrown around) alleged statements attributed to Sanger regarding eugenics. Margaret Sanger did support the eugenic objective of promoting favorable genetic characteristics in ways she hoped would accelerate human evolution in positive ways, in the years before such ideas were discredited by Adolf Hitler's version, which was rooted in race-based "Aryan supremacy." In the years after Hitler's perversion of the concept, eugenics fell into appropriate disfavor.

Moreover, they assert that Planned Parenthood today is hypocritical because the modern organization supports the right of women to choose to abort unwanted pregnancies, but cite statements attributed to its founder, Margaret Sanger, that seem to indicate opposition to abortion. We must remember that Sanger operated in a time when abortion was outlawed everywhere, widely held to be a disreputable, immoral and illegal choice, and she was able to correctly note, for anyone opposed to abortion, that the birth control options she promoted (also held in disrepute in those early days) provided the most effective means of preventing the unwanted pregnancies that motivate a choice to abort in the first place.

But here is the funny thing: there is a certain irony for someone who claims to be opposed to abortion to denigrate someone who they are asserting was, like themselves, opposed to abortion. Huh? There is a certain irony in someone alleging terrible things about someone and then noting that, by the way, the person they are denigrating agrees more with themselves than with the organization they founded as it evolved into its current incarnation of today.

The fact is that Planned Parenthood has evolved from the organization Margaret Sanger founded, into the organization it is today. Whatever the beliefs of its founder, in a different time and place, in a different cultural milieu, the organization today is pro-choice and, while not primarily a provider of abortions, does support the right of women to terminate unwanted pregnancies as a viable option for women who make that choice.

Planned Parenthood today offers a full range of medical and reproductive services for women and also for men. The beliefs and opinions of its founder are not relevant to the moral, legal and religious issues surrounding abortion and the rights of women to control their own personal and private medical and reproductive choices.

Federal Funding of Planned Parenthood and abortion

One of the criticism often raised against Planned Parenthood and abortion is that federal tax dollars should not be used to cover a practice that many object to on moral grounds, though the same critics rarely accept the inverse of that argument is applied to the military choice to invade another country or to allow lower taxes on the investment gains of millionaires, no matter how many people object to those policies on moral grounds.

The argument goes that even if people have the right to abort an unwanted pregnancy, they should be responsible for their own medical expenses.

There are several problems with this line of argument.

The first is that abortion is a medical procedure. Federal tax dollars are involved in funding many medical procedures and to arbitrarily discriminate against women's medical services because some people object to them, while covering blood transfusions that Jehovah's Witnesses object to (or any medical treatment at all that Seventh Day Adventists object to) is outright discrimination based on gender.

But there is a more grievous error involved here.

The entire premise is false. There is no federal funding of abortion, and has not been since 1976.

As noted earlier, in the section about the legal aspects of abortion and how denial of funding is a strategy used by those opposed to women's reproductive rights without a direct prohibition on abortion that would be unconstitutional, the Hyde Amendment was passed on September 30, 1976. It was introduced by Henry Hyde, a rabid anti-abortion extremist congressman and self-proclaimed moral arbiter from Illinois. This was the same Congressman Hyde who was one of the Congressional leaders and judgmental moralists who brought impeachment charges against President Bill Clinton on moral grounds, for engaging in oral sex.

Congressman Hyde, typical of so many judgmental moralizing hypocrites, was subsequently forced to step down when he himself was caught in adultery. The moral hypocrisy and double standard astounds.

But the fact remains: since 1976, there has been no use of Federal tax dollars to fund abortion operations in the United States. Yet the myth persists and campaigns to defund other non-abortion services are threatened by the persistence of such misinformation.

The fact is that Planned Parenthood receives no federal funding for the relatively small proportion of abortions it provides. It does receive, appropriately, funding for other preventive and therapeutic medical services including cancer screenings, mammograms, birth control, vasectomies, prevention and treatments of sexually-transmitted diseases and so much more.

As for allegations sometimes raised that Planed Parenthood takes its federal funding and then just hands it back to supportive political candidates or engages in other political activity, this is also false. No such political funding or campaign contributions come from Planned Parenthood. Such allegations confuse Planned Parenthood with Planned Parenthood Action Fund, a separate but affiliated political action committee which does engage in political activity to promote the institutional values and activities against the barrage of political attacks constantly levied against it.

Some may question the ethical legitimacy of having an affiliated political action committee, and question the extent to which these organizations are really separate.

No secret is made of the fact that the two organizations are affiliated and aligned. The importance of maintaining separate organizations is to provide a clear mechanism by which donors can ensure that if they want to donate to a medical and social services non-profit they can do so knowing their contributions will be used only for that purpose, and if they wish to promote public policies and candidates in support of that organization and its services, they can also do that knowingly.

It is all open, transparent and empowering to those who wish to contribute, to ensure that their contributions will be used only as intended.

Anti-choice conservatives love to wield simplistic slogans and cheap attacks, but when examined in grater detail, they do not hold up. Often the points they make, when examined at deeper than a superficial level, end up arguing against the conclusions they were trying to promote.

Complex issues of social, personal and public morality can rarely be reduced to a size that will fit on the bumper of a car.